Natural *alternatives* to Dieting

Dr Marilyn Glenville, PhD is a nutritional therapist, psychologist, broadcaster and author of the internationally best-selling *Natural Alternatives to HRT*. She obtained her doctorate from Cambridge University. She is the Chair of the Governing Council for the British Association of Nutritional Therapists and the Chair of Foresight (the association for the promotion of pre-conceptual care) as well as a scientific adviser to the Society for the Promotion of Nutritional Therapy.

For more than twenty years Dr Glenville has practised nutritional therapy in the UK and the USA. She has had several papers published in scientific journals, frequently advises health professionals and often lectures at academic conferences held at the Medical Society and the Royal College of Physicians. As a respected authority on women's healthcare, she gives regular talks on radio and has often appeared on television and in the press.

Dr Glenville has been officially appointed by the Ministry of Agriculture, Food and Fisheries to be an observer with the Expert Group (which advises safe levels of vitamins and minerals in food supplements). She is also the Chair of the steering group for the Nutritional Therapy Council, instigated by the Government to set national occupational standards for Nutritional Therapy in the UK.

She practises from four private clinics in London, Kent, and Sussex including the Hale Clinic.

Natural
alternatives
to
Dieting

Marilyn Glenville

NEW MILLENNIUM BOOKS
Vancouver

First published in Canada in 1999 by
New Millennium Books
8036 Enterprise Street
Burnaby, BC V5A 1V7
T: (604)b 415-2444   F: 9604) 415-3444

10 9 8 7 6 5 4 3

ISBN 1 85626 317 7

Text © 1999 Marilyn Glenville
Illustration © 1999 Roland Ungoed-Thomas
Recipes pages 157-179 © Wendy Hutton and Jane Frank

Marilyn Glenville is hereby identified as the author of this
work in accordance with Section 77 of the Copyright, Designs
and Patents Act 1988

A CIP catalogue record for this title is
available from the British Library

Typeset by SX Composing DTP, Rayleigh, Essex
Printed and bound in Wales by WBC Book Manufacturers

The contents of this book are for information only and are intended to assist
readers in identifying symptoms and conditions they may be experiencing. The
book is not intended to be a substitute for taking proper medical advice and
should not be relied upon in this way. Always consult a qualified doctor or
health practitioner. The author and publisher cannot accept responsibility for
illness arising out of the failure to seek medical advice from a doctor.

What people have said about
Natural alternatives to HRT

'I highly recommend this book to all women as an invaluable life guide'.
Liz Earle, author and broadcaster

'A great book – I particularly liked its passion and its practicality.'
Dr Penny Stanway, author

'This is a truly ground-breaking book and is not to be missed. It shows there really are genuinely natural ways to enjoy good health right through the menopause, ensuring choice, control and freedom for future years.'
International Journal of Alternative and Complementary Medicine.

'Natural Alternatives to HRT throws down the gauntlet to conventional thinking... this book is all about choices and arms readers with the knowledge that will help them manage their bodies and enjoy a balanced and positive life without having to resort to pills.'
The Good Times

To Kriss — with all my love

Contents

Acknowledgements

The help and support of many people including my family, friends and associates have made this book possible.

I would particularly like to thank Pamela Townsend for her expertise in making this book coherent and clear. Dr Penny Stanway was again extremely helpful in reviewing the draft and her medical expertise and opinion were invaluable. A very special thank you goes to Wendy Hutton and Jane Frank for their superb contribution of the delicious recipes as well as to Olivers Wholefood Store. My thanks also to Kate Oldfield, my editor at Kyle Cathie, for her continuing encouragement and to Kyle and her excellent team for their understanding that this book needed to be written. Thanks also to Teresa Hale of the Hale Clinic and Mr Mehta of the Nutri Centre. Thanks also go to Linda McVan, my practice manager, and to all the staff who keep my practice running smoothly. Their ability to work as a team and to have a sense of humour has been invaluable.

My love goes to my husband Kriss and my children Matthew, Leonard and Chantell, who are ever supportive and understanding.

I would also like to express my deep appreciation to Yehudi Gordon, consultant gynaecologist and obstetrician, and all the staff at Viveka. This is a conventional medical practice with the open-mindedness to incorporate a holistic approach to women's healthcare. Nutrition is seen as a vital part of this practice and I value working with Yehudi and his colleagues.

Exploding the diet myths

Are these statements true or false?

1. If you eat less you will lose weight.
2. Eating any form of fat is unhealthy and must be avoided.
3. Snacking between meals will make you put on weight.
4. Foods that are labelled 'low fat' will help you slim.
5. You must stick to a reduced diet to become thinner.
6. If you skip breakfast you'll lose weight because it reduces your daily calorie intake.
7. You must exercise at a high intensity to lose fat.
8. Margarine is better for you than butter.

ALL of the above are false.

Introduction

Eating to live

If you're fed up with dieting, you're in good company. In fact you are a member, along with millions of other people, of what is probably the largest club in the world. The largest club with the unhappiest membership. To fail at weight control can be devastating. At the very least it is tiresome and boring, but the effects can be even more severe than that. Failed dieters often suffer depression, lack of confidence and damaged self-esteem.

So what's the alternative?

What more can you do? You've read all the articles about weight control, tried every diet under the sun, maybe even joined a slimming club and, perhaps for a few heady weeks or months, you reached your target weight. But once you stop dieting and return to your old eating habits you find that the weight piles on again. This is because you are probably eating the same food which was making you put on weight in the first place. The inescapable truth is that diets, as we've known them, don't work – at least not for long.

It is easy to try one diet, then another and another in the quest to lose weight but, before you realise what's happening, you've become what is known as a yo-yo dieter with your weight going up and down. Apart from being disappointing and demoralising, yo-yoing is unhealthy because it distorts your attitude to food and steers you away from a normal eating pattern.

This yo-yo effect fosters feelings of anger and resentment as food becomes the 'enemy' which you should not submit to. In the extreme, this has led to a number of eating disorders such as anorexia and bulimia, particularly among women, but men (especially teenage boys) can also be affected.

Women, and also men these days, face a lot of pressure to look good.

Every time we turn on the television or watch a film we see constant reminders of beautiful body-shape. There are endless magazine articles about weight loss, image make-overs, make-up, plastic surgery and anti-ageing creams. The result is pressure, pressure, pressure.

The diet business in the UK has an annual turnover of £6 billion, having grown by nearly 200% in the last eight years. Slimming pills, replacement drinks, gimmicks like fat-attraction pills, lo-cal this, lo-fat that, are big profit earners. One wouldn't be too cynical to assume that the last thing the diet industry wants is for people to diet and then stay slim.

However, despite the huge diet industry and our collective efforts to lose weight we are actually getting bigger and bigger. According to government figures published in 1998, half the population is classified as overweight and the obesity figures have doubled in the past five years. Some 16% of women and 13% of men in the UK are now obese, which means they are approximately 20% heavier than they should be. The November 1998 edition of the *Pharmaceutical Times* talked about obesity now being an epidemic in the developed countries. With the rising obesity figures and the fact that 57% of men and 48% of women carry excess weight, the UK has a weight problem which is spiralling out of control.

We are more sedentary now, and that is a contributing factor, but the main reason for the rise in obesity is the change in the type of food we eat. This has affected our health in general and our weight in particular. Nowadays we eat more refined food, more convenience food, more junk food and at least 30% more fat than we did in the early 1900s.

The fact that we actually take in fewer calories today than we did at the beginning of the century challenges the traditional view that we only put on weight if we eat too many calories. If calories alone were the reason we put on weight, then we would all be thin.

Researchers have found that fat and thin people eat roughly the same number of calories but fat people eat a different type of food from thin people.

This book will explain which foods are better for you and introduce you to a way of eating which is delicious and nourishing while allowing your weight to reduce naturally over time and then remain stable. It will also help you to banish food cravings and say goodbye to food-related mood swings. It will advise you on shopping for food, preparing meals to eat at home with your family and will also encourage you to eat out in restaurants sometimes and have a normal social life! It's all about discovering a way of eating that you can maintain and enjoy.

This isn't just another diet book?

The information this book contains is gimmick-free and works. It gives you a new way of thinking about food where you'll understand that the body needs to work in harmony with what you feed it. Any imbalance in the body's functions can have far-reaching effects.

This book will also advise on exercise not just as an aid to weight loss but also to benefit your general health. It will show that exercise can be woven into your everyday routine in ways that you might not have thought of before.

If, after following the advice given, you still have trouble losing weight, you will also learn about the role of nutritional therapy in weight loss and tests that are available to identify health problems which are affecting your weight.

Prepare yourself for a major life change and start eating to live rather than living to eat. You'll be amazed at the difference.

CHAPTER 1

Why diets don't work

Dieting is a losing battle. As you reduce your food intake as part of a diet to lose weight, your body puts itself on 'famine alert'. It gets the impression that food is scarce and therefore it slows down your metabolism to get the best use of the small amount of food it is receiving. If, for example, you crash diet for a week and then go back to your normal pattern of eating, you will be consuming your normal diet with a slower metabolism which means you will regain the lost weight and maybe even put on new weight.

Eat little and often

With most diets, you will lose only a small amount of fat before your body's fat protection mechanism swings into action. In this state of famine, your body will hold on to fat, break down muscle and lose water. But, if you eat little and often, your body 'knows' that food is plentiful. It doesn't need to store any excess in case there is a shortage and it can keep your metabolism at a good level.

What is a calorie?

A calorie, in scientific terms, is a unit of heat and is the energy-producing property of food. The idea has been that if the number of calories going into your body is less than the calories being used up by bodily activity and exercise, then you will lose weight. Nowadays, though, we know that the type of calorie is also an important factor in this equation and we need to consider its source – whether it's from fat, protein or carbohydrate.

Fat or energy

Food can be converted into fat or energy. You can either store what you eat, which means you will probably put on weight, or you can use it as you expend energy in life's activities. Whether food is burned or stored is determined by a number of chemical reactions which are activated by enzymes, which in turn are dependent upon vitamins and minerals. However, not all types of foods are easy to convert into energy and when their conversion is not possible the body stores them as fat, which is a sign that it is not metabolising the food properly.

Crash diets

When you go on a diet your body cannot distinguish between a diet and a journey through the desert. It doesn't know whether the small portion of food you have just given it will be the last food it's going to get for a long while. So its defence mechanisms step in and it holds on to any food it comes across.

A little bit won't hurt

Imagine that you have been dieting for a couple of days and a friend brings you a cake. You decide to take a taste of the cake on the basis that 'a little bit won't hurt'. Once you begin to eat you find you can't stop and before you realise it you've eaten half the cake! Instantly damaging emotions such as guilt and anger take over. But your response was a simple and quite natural, bio-logical urge. Your body prepared itself for the possibility that the cake might be a last chance to stock up. It triggered into action a cocktail of chemicals which are programmed to act on your behalf in terms of survival but not in terms of your waistline.

Quite simply, trying to lose weight rapidly by crash dieting is against your body's programming. It requires you to be in a biologically unnatural state where energy intake is less than energy expenditure. Your mind and body quickly hear alarm bells and resort to strong tactics to persuade you to eat normally.

Listen to your hunger urges

Instead of crash dieting try working in harmony with your body and its nat-ural urges of hunger – you will be able to eat well, stay healthy and maintain your ideal body weight.

A study published by the *American Journal of Clinical Nutrition* in 1996 showed that keeping our weight stable over long periods of time is linked with the best health. It is fine to lose excess weight but the problem is what is termed 'weight cycling', where weight is lost, then gained, then lost again and so on. Studies have shown that weight variations caused by yo-yo diet-ing may be associated with health problems such as increased risk of diabetes, high blood pressure and increased mortality risk from coronary heart disease.[1]

Women have more fat cells than men

A man has 26 billion fat cells, or adipocytes, in his body while the female average is 35 billion. Fat comprises 27% of an average woman's total body-weight but for a man comprises only 15%. There are biological reasons for women to have more fat on their bodies than men. Fat is essential for reproduction and therefore nature keeps fat stored on the female frame just in case a pregnancy begins. It is also necessary for ovulation – it's known that girls don't begin to menstruate until their bodies are composed of at least 17% fat. Some women who have taken dieting to the extreme over a long period of time have found that they couldn't conceive. Athletes, gymnasts and anorexics can also find, albeit for different reasons, that their periods will stop if their body fat stores fall too low.

A study published in the medical journal *The Lancet* in 1998 showed that men prefer women to be curvaceous – curves signify fertility and health which men find attractive. The message from the author of the study, Dr Tovee of Newcastle University's Psychology Department, is that 'women are much better putting on too much weight than losing too much weight'.

Weight and the menopause

As the ovaries produce less and less oestrogen during the menopause, body fat becomes an alternative manufacturing plant for this vital hormone: oestrogen helps the older woman combat the risk of osteoporosis. Fat produces oestrogen all our lives, which is why low- and no-fat diets, so often recommended to slimmers, are a big mistake for women throughout their lives. During and post menopause, body fat is even more vital to good health and it can be quite natural to be a few kilograms (half a stone) over the pre-menopausal weight.

However, the balance is delicate: too much body fat post menopause and you run the risk of having too much oestrogen in your body – a state known as oestrogen dominance – and that has health risks, such as breast cancer, attached to it.

Not surprisingly it is now believed that being the right weight for height is very important in ensuring the post-menopausal woman has enough fat for the production of oestrogen. The body mass index (BMI) which is explained more fully in Chapter 5 is the best way to determine this. Several studies have shown that BMI is a reliable indicator of osteoporosis risk.[2] One demonstrated that women aged 45 to 59 who had suffered fractures had an average BMI of 22.5, while those without fractures had an average BMI of 25.3.[3] As the BMI falls, bone density declines even in the absence of fractures. It seems that losing a significant amount of weight quickly may be particularly relevant to loss of bone mass.

Nature may have tipped the scales against women in their fight against fat but has also protected itself from the vanities of the female by making it harder for women to lose weight than men.

When dieting becomes a way of life

When you begin to diet it's not always easy to know when to stop. Dieting becomes a way of life and it's possible to feel 'naked' or 'unprotected' when you aren't on one. This mindset can make you set unrealistic goals. To aim to shed every gram of excess fat is to make the hurdle too high to jump, not just in terms of willpower, but, as we've just discussed, in health terms too.

We can't all be a size 10

Of course to be obese is dangerous. To be over-weight to the point of possibly damaging your health is daft and must be tackled, but how many of us are naturally a size 10? For a start not all of us have the bone structure and general body frame for that – in fact the average size for women in the UK is 16. As nature has already determined your size, trying to be any smaller is probably a waste of time.

An interesting study[4] looked at a random sample of 1,053 women aged 30-74 and found that only 25% were satisfied with their weight. A staggering 71% of the women wanted to be thinner and yet 73% of them were at their normal weight. Many attempted dieting even when they were at their medically correct weight.

Thin v. curvaceous – a dictate of fashion?

A desire for a sylph-like body is by no means universal, nor has it always been with us. Big women in Fiji and Arabia, for example, are considered to be attractive, while the West's greatest ever sex symbol, Marilyn Monroe, was a size 16. Time was when curves like hers were highly desirable, but now, with waif-like supermodels to emulate, women expect to be so thin that millions remain on a permanent diet. Of course, there are health risks in being excessively overweight, but it seems that our society has now swung too far the other way, with many women literally starving themselves to some extent every day.

A history of dieting

All diets purport to help us lose weight, but if they worked, why are there still so many unhappy overweight women? The methods people have used to lose weight over the years fall roughly into three categories:

1. Popular diets recommended by friends and advertisements
2. Surgery
3. Use of drugs

The following will explain the theory behind each method and analyse how successful they have been in terms of weight loss and being healthy.

POPULAR DIETS

You may recognise, or indeed have tried, some of the following popular diets:

Very Low Calorie Diets (VLCDs)

Very low calorie diets are diets which are based on restricting calories to sometimes fewer than 500 a day. This is achieved by using complete meal replacements. Some of these very low calorie diets provide the back-up support of a counsellor but for the majority you have to manage on your own. Replacement meals take the form of milk shakes, soups and bars. The replacement meals are designed to give the British recommended daily allowance (RDA) of viatamins and minerals.

Verdict

These diets require a lot of willpower and by their nature are very boring. The weight loss can be dramatic but in almost starving yourself you can lose not just fat but muscle as well, which is medically unwise. To lose heart muscle, for example is potentially fatal.

Many of these diets don't change long established bad eating patterns nor do they offer help once the diet is over. Also, as the body is being starved, it will automatically lower the metabolic rate in order to protect itself. So as the person returns to their normal eating pattern with a slower metabolism, more weight can be gained.

There are a number of meal substitute diets on the market and some can be purchased over shop counters. All VLCDs involve the replacement of one or two ordinary meals a day. They can work well for women who are busy and they do contain the RDA of vitamins and minerals but should be used with caution.

F Plan

F stands for 'fibre' and this diet, introduced in the early 1980s, was based on the idea that high-fibre food passes through our system so fast that the body doesn't have the chance to absorb all the calories from it. It was believed that the more fibre there was in our diet, the more calories would be excreted and the greater would be our weight loss. The dieter was given the recipe for a special high-fibre muesli, called 'fibre filler', which provided 15g (½oz) of dietary fibre daily.

Verdict

Apart from being boring, the main criticism of the F Plan has been that it makes everything pass through the body too quickly, thereby reducing the absorption of valuable nutrients.

Food combining

This is an eating regime where protein and starch (carbohydrate) are eaten at separate meals based on the belief that these two foods need different enzymes to be digested effectively. It is said that if they are eaten together the resulting undigested food is stored firstly in the intestines resulting in fermentation which leads to bloating and flatulence, then, if not properly digested and used as energy, it will be stored as fat.

The rules of the regime are:

- Don't mix starchy foods with proteins
- Eat fruit on its own
- Don't have milk with either starch or protein

Rules that are often added to the above include:

- High-fat dairy foods should not be eaten more than once in five days

- Cut down on wheat products
- Pulses (such as lentils) should be avoided because they in themselves combine protein and starch

Verdict

The theory behind this regime does not seem to have been proven scientific-ally and yet there are people who feel the regime has helped with digestive problems (which in turn has helped them to lose weight). These people often choose to stay permanently on this regime. Critics often focus on a number of points including: eating lean meat without fibre can slow down its passage through the gut; food combining works only because it restricts food intake and helps the person become more aware of what they are eating.

A theory based on the Glycaemic Index (see Chapter 2) suggests that we do need to eat protein and carbohydrate together.

High protein/no carbohydrate

This kind of diet was popular in the 1970s and was based on eating lots of protein such as meat and eggs but no carbohydrate such as bread, pasta, rice or potatoes. Initial weight loss was good – up to 6kg (1 stone) in the first week but, unfortunately, it was water loss not fat.

When the body is starved of carbohydrates it looks for energy in its glycogen stores and because 4g (0.14oz) of water cling to every gram of glycogen, it is possible to lose a lot of weight very quickly. It is only when the glycogen stores are depleted that the body starts to dissolve the fat. This happens very slowly so it seems that the diet has stopped working. These pro-tein only diets can cause an abnormal metabolic state called ketosis because there is not enough carbohydrate stored in the liver for the body to use.

Verdict

A difficulty with these high protein ketogenic diets is that they can bring about changes in the fat cells causing them to accumulate even more fat when the person comes off the diet. They have also created problems with mood changes, such as tension and irritability, resulting in cravings for carbohydrate-rich foods and fatty snacks.

Interestingly, when a diet is high in carbohydrates and low in protein, brain serotonin (the 'feel-good' hormone) levels have increased, thereby improving mood and appetite. In a study of 40 obese women with a long history of yo-yo dieting, a diet of 1,400 calories derived from a high carbo-hydrate/low protein diet gave them fewer cravings and better overall moods after several weeks compared to those on the 1,400 calorie high protein/low carbohydrate diet.[5] Also, those on the high carbohydrate diet lost significantly more weight than those on the high protein diet.

Hip and thigh-type diets

These concentrate on being very low fat, sometimes no fat, which is a dangerous concept and one we will return to in Chapter 3. The dieter is asked not to eat fat including oils, nuts (except chestnuts), seeds, oily fish, cheese (except cottage cheese), milk (except skimmed), egg yolk (egg white is acceptable), crisps and avocados and to remove all fat and skin from poultry.

Verdict

The reduction of fat in specific areas of the body (such as hips and thighs) has never been proved possible, but these diets do seem to help with general weight loss. It's true that we generally eat too much fat – on average between 50 and 60% of our calorie intake is from fat. Logic tells us that if we cut out all fat we will lose weight, but at what cost to our health? Certain fats, known as essential fatty acids (EFAs) are, as their name suggests, essential for our health and it is unwise to go on a diet that eliminates them along with all the non-essential fats such as saturated fat. The body cannot produce essential fats, so the only source of these is from what we eat. Totally fat-free diets have resulted in joint stiffness, skin problems and mood swings.

Essential fats are a vital component of every human cell and the body needs them to:

- insulate nerve cells
- keep skin and arteries supple
- balance hormones
- keep us warm

Women who have made sure they are getting enough EFAs – either in their food or taken as supplements – have found relief from benign breast disease and 'lumpy' breasts. EFAs can also increase metabolic rate, which in turn stimulates fat burn-off and increased weight loss. A good intake of EFAs is important too for those suffering with skin conditions such as eczema.

The 'skinny' diet or heart diet

This diet became quite a sensation as it was faxed around America in 1997 like a chain letter. The regime involves unlimited bowls of soup (made from spring onions, green peppers, celery, onion soup mix and canned tomatoes), supplemented with different foods on successive days.

Food plan

Day One	Soup and fruit
Day Two	Soup and vegetables with buttered baked potato
Day Three	Soup, fruit and vegetables
Day Four	Soup, eight bananas and skimmed milk
Day Five	Soup, beef and tomatoes
Day Six	Same as Day Five
Day Seven	Soup, brown rice and vegetables

Verdict

The diet is only to be followed for one week and, while it can be boring, it does effect a weight loss. However it doesn't change eating habits which are the key to sustained weight loss. The dieter is left high and dry at the end of the seven days with no guidance on post-diet eating.

Few foods diet

This diet comes and goes with different fads and trends. It usually concentrates on one or only a few foods. Popular versions have been the grapefruit only diet and there is another which allowed up to six hard boiled eggs and six tomatoes a day.

Verdict

As with meal replacement diets, these take the thinking out of what to eat. The diets will be deficient in essential vitamins and minerals and of course lack any variety which will make them difficult to stick to.

SURGERY

The following are rather unusual, and at times dangerous, ways of trying to lose weight:

Jaw wiring

This was an early weight loss idea whereby the jaw was wired so that no solids, only liquids, could be eaten. It is still an available option. Once the weight loss is achieved the wiring is removed. Sadly, it has seldom worked in the long term as lost weight is usually regained once the jaws are unwired. The dieter has not learned a new way of eating, so a return to 'old' eating habits can cause quite a rapid gain in weight.

Stomach stapling

This is a popular surgical technique where, under anaesthetic, the stomach is literally stapled to make its volume much smaller. The dieter feels full more quickly and therefore stops eating sooner. Unfortunately it doesn't always work because the stomach can be stretched by overeating even when stapled. The staples can also burst, which requires major surgery.

Lap band

This is the newest technique and involves a surgical procedure whereby a giant silicone band is placed inside the body, around the stomach. It works on the same principle as stomach stapling in that it reduces the room for food in the stomach. It is said to be a less painful operation than stomach stapling and the patient goes home after just three days in hospital. As with any surgical procedure, the benefits must always be weighed against the risks which accompany any use of anaesthetics, and which are greater in cases of obesity.

Liposuction

This is where the fat is literally sucked out from under the skin while the dieter is fully conscious. The operation is very occasionally lethal and is not recommended. It is usually only performed around the hip and thigh areas – it would be even more dangerous to suck out fat from the abdomen due to the risk of damaging internal organs. As with any surgery, there can be side effects such as infection and numbness in the area. Women have also complained of being left with baggy skin which has been excessive in some cases.

Stomach balloon

This is a keyhole technique whereby a doctor working with a small camera inserts a silicone balloon into the stomach via the mouth and then proceeds to inflate it with water. The balloon stays in place for up to six months before being burst and removed via the mouth. As with stomach stapling and the lap band, this makes the volume of the stomach much smaller, so less food is required to feel full.

Stomach by-pass

An even more drastic and newer surgical operation than those described above involves stapling the stomach and creating a shortcut round the upper digestive tract and by-passing 1.5m (5ft) of small intestine. This technique reduces the number of calories absorbed and also makes the person sick if they try to over-indulge. Side effects can be liver and kidney damage because of the interference with digestion.

Removal of lower ribs

The lower ribs are surgically removed so that the person can attain an hour-glass figure. Along with the other plastic surgery she has had done, the singer and actor Cher underwent this procedure to change her body shape and give the appearance of being slimmer.

Weight loss patch

This patch originated in America but is now widely available. It contains Fucus, a type of seaweed found off the Atlantic coasts of France and Ireland. Seaweed naturally contains high levels of iodine which is a mineral that can help to regulate metabolism. Kelp, another seaweed, has also been used for weight loss in the past. Two thirds of our body's iodine is in the thyroid, the gland that controls metabolism. Traditionally, herbalists have used *Fucus vesiculosus* (bladder wrack) as an oral medicine to help those who are over-weight. When the dose is administered using a patch it is difficult to know how much iodine is absorbed through the skin.

Weight loss worms

Around the turn of the century, dieters could purchase a tapeworm, neatly encapsulated for easy swallowing. In theory, the worm would gobble up all the extra food you ate and so keep you slim. There are apparently still ads for weight loss worms on the Internet but you are not advised to try them!

Can surgery keep weight off?

None of the surgical techniques outlined (or the worms!) helps someone to retrain their eating patterns and keep their weight under control.

USE OF DRUGS

The desperate dieter has sometimes been prescribed drugs by a doctor or bought over-the-counter dieting aids. Drugs have traditionally worked in one of two ways.

1. By increasing brain levels of serotonin:
These drugs work as an anti-depressant, boosting the brain chemical serotonin which curbs appetite and lifts mood. Two of the most widely prescribed used to be dexfenfluramine and fenfluramine, but they had many side effects including:

- dry mouth
- nausea
- dizziness
- drowsiness
- nervousness
- headaches

They were also found to be linked with primary pulmonary hypertension where a heart and lung transplant was needed. In this potentially fatal condition the blood pressure in the arteries feeding the lungs is abnormally high. In some cases, the blood can barely get through, putting the heart under massive strain. Thankfully, these drugs have now been withdrawn from the market. (You'll learn in Chapter 2 how carbohydrates can increase serotonin levels, decreasing your appetite naturally and lifting your mood.)

2. By stimulating the central nervous system

These amphetamine-based drugs work by reducing hunger and food intake and stimulating the stress response. Some can be addictive as they give a feeling of euphoria. But side effects of phentermine, one of the most widely used, include:

- restlessness
- dry mouth
- high blood pressure
- hallucinations

Phentermine needs a GP's prescription and supervision. Unfortunately some slimming clinics have been selling the drugs without proper scrutiny of the dieter's medical history and without the vital on-going supervision. The lax control of these drugs has also contributed to an illegal black market with patients' health being placed at risk.

'Wonder' drugs

The latest 'wonder' drug, available in Britain from September 1998 is Xenical, destined, it was claimed, to become as popular as Viagra.

Xenical contains orlistat, the first of a new breed of drugs which, working in the gut, actually reduces the capacity of the body to absorb fat into the blood stream. Instead of being digested, the fat is excreted. The drug prevents absorption of about one-third of fat, about 600 calories a day, which should lead to a weight loss of about 450g (1lb) a week. Because excess fat goes straight through the body, the dieters are asked to eat a low-fat diet otherwise they can get diarrhoea. This seems a contradiction in itself. Other known side effects include:

- anal leakage
- flatulence
- bowel pain

Xenical is available on prescription only from a doctor and is intended for people with very serious over-weight problems whose progress can be monitored by their doctor. It is feared that, as with other slimming pills, a black market trade might develop which would result in dieters not having proper medical supervision. It is also possible that, as it is such a new drug, not all side-effects are yet known – there has already been some concern in the US that it may increase the risk of breast cancer. It may also carry with it the same problems as the fat-free fat (see below), in that it might prevent the absorption of vitamins A, D, E and K which are fat soluble and important for health.

Appetite-suppressing chewing gum

This new gum, developed in 1998 by a Swiss company, contains as its main ingredient chromium picolinate. A number of research papers have focused on chromium as an effective aid for weight loss. Chromium is needed for the metabolism of fats and the regulation of blood sugar levels. The gum is said to be mint-flavoured and sugar-free which suggests that artificial sweeteners may have been added instead. The American Cancer Society has found that people who regularly use artificial sweeteners tend to gain weight, not lose it. The sweeteners can also slow down the digestive process and increase appetite. Chewing triggers the flow of digestive juices and can increase the feeling of hunger, which could urge you to eat more than you need. However, chromium is important as a food supplement and ways of taking it are discussed in Chapter 7.

Fat-free fat

This is a product, going by the name of Olestra, which is widely used in America and could be introduced elsewhere. It is put into foods such as crisps and chips and has the effect of binding six or eight fatty acids to sugar molecules. This changes the fats' chemistry so they are no longer susceptible to the stomach's digestive enzymes and therefore pass through the body unabsorbed.

The problem is this may also affect our absorption of fat-soluble vitamins such as A, D, E and K plus the group of nutrients knows as carotenoids, which may have a vital role in the prevention of cancer and heart disease. To get round this problem the company has now added extra vitamins to the zero-fat foods.

Normal fat is made of three fatty acids – called triglycerides – and they must be broken down by enzymes before they can be digested. Zero-fats are synthetic and are not broken down by these enzymes. Users of foods containing zero-fats have suffered side effects, including:

- intestinal cramping
- flatulence
- loose bowels

The exact reasons for these side effects is unknown.

A study of 76 people carried out in 1998 by the gastroenterology department of Addenbrooke's Hospital in Cambridge and published in the *British Journal of Nutrition* shows that people who ate Olestra had lower levels of the fat soluble carotenoids and lower levels of vitamin E, a fat soluble vitamin. Thirty per cent of the group also suffered significant bowel irritations.

Fat absorbers and fat attraction pills

Purchased mainly in pill form from health stores, these take the idea of binding agents one step further. They provide fibre but supposedly 'grab' undigested fat in the intestine and then carry it out of the body. They are made from chitosan, a powder made from finely ground prawns, crabs, or other shellfish. Manufacturers claim it binds with fats, causing them to pass through the gut without being absorbed. They also claim that it soaks up lipids and bile to prevent them from being absorbed into the blood stream. The problem is that it is just as likely to dispense with necessary unsaturated fats and fat soluble vitamins as with the unnecessary saturated ones. Apparently the substance has been used for around 30 years in water purification plants, where it is spread over the surface of the water to absorb oil, grease and toxic waste. (For more on the role of fibre in helping to lose weight, see Chapter 3.)

Why risk taking drugs?

All drugs carry some risk of side effects and unless you are obese, or unless you have a specific medical reason for having to take them, why take the risk? After all, you have to come off them at some stage and they will have done nothing to help you rid your eating regime of bad habits. If you decide you must have the support of a drug then be sure to go to your GP. Don't buy on the black market, from friends, or from slimming clinics unless they thoroughly check your medical history.

You would be far better off learning to eat properly and, with the help of this book, you can do it!

Food adulteration to aid weight control

Research is ongoing into food adulteration. A joint collaboration between the Medical Research Council and the food industry is looking at the possibility of altering the structure of our food so that it makes us feel happier and eat less.

When we cut down the amount of food we eat we reduce the level of a naturally occurring essential amino acid call tryptophan which is involved in the production of serotonin, one of the brain chemicals which help govern our moods (see Chapter 2).

Serotonin is found naturally in:

- dairy products
- meat
- fish
- turkey
- bananas
- dried dates
- peanuts

The idea now is to add tryptophan artificially to foods such as biscuits. Where will it all end? Our choices as consumers will be affected – we won't know what we are eating or what effect it may have on us. We now have fluoride in our water supply; why not also add aspirin to prevent us from getting headaches or birth control pills to keep the population down!

Tryptophan could, however, have a place as a food supplement and this is discussed in Chapter 7.

Take control of your own body

Dieters will constantly look for a crutch to lean on, an outside influence to boost their own, quite natural, flagging willpower. The more we diet and want gimmicks to help us lose weight, the more big business will try to give them to us. They make money while we fail. They provide the next fad and we pay for it.

In one survey, the Advertising Standards Authority found that 80% of the advertisements for slimming remedies made unsubstantiated claims, and many of the products were not effective. The time is definitely here to take matters into your own hands. Take control of your own body, your own diet, your own eating pattern and your own appetite.

What controls appetite?

The hypothalamus in the brain masterminds the whole process, but other factors count too. Emotions, for example, play a large role. Eating when we are bored, stressed or unhappy is not a response to hunger but to a psychological need for comfort.

Research has also found that your appetite is influenced not only by the quantity of food eaten, but also the type. When you have eaten enough, signals are sent to the brain which then stops you from eating any more. Carbohydrates and proteins are good at sending signals and are much stronger appetite-suppressants than fats – like ice cream or chocolate. Likewise it's signals from the brain that make you eat. You eat for energy. When your store of energy is running low your brain sends out a signal to eat for fuel.

It sounds simple and it should be, but once you start putting on excess weight the whole subject of food and appetite becomes a lot more complicated. Nature's delicate balance becomes distorted when some days you eat healthily but others you stock up on junk. There may be times when you're too full to finish a salad but have room for a dessert and other times when you have overpowering cravings for certain foods. These rather abnormal eating patterns are often associated with the menopause and menstrual cycle.

Make food part of life, not an obsession

You've got to eat to live and, as long as the overall trend is sensible, inconsistencies in what you eat can be accommodated by your body. The prevailing obsession with food (all too often with unhealthy food) causes many of the problems that over-weight people have to struggle with today.

Fat distribution and heart disease

Research at London's St. Thomas's Hospital in 1997 revealed some new and extremely interesting information.[6] The tests were carried out on 350 sets of middle-aged twins over a three year period. It was discovered that women with a big tummy have a higher risk of heart disease, high blood pressure and diabetes. This is because the type of fat which gathers around the waist constantly breaks down and circulates in the blood.

Researchers also found that 60% of body fat in women over 50 is caused by genetic make-up. By comparing identical and non-identical twins, they found that the distribution of fat on the body rather than its quantity was the key to predicting future health. According to Dr Tim Spector, Director of the Twins Research Unit at St. Thomas's, the study also showed that because fat tends to build up around a man's waist (rather than his bottom) men suffer more heart disease than women. Pear-shaped women with large bottoms and thighs not only suffered less heart disease and diabetes than 'straight up and down' women but also had better blood pressure.

How does your weight affect your health?

If the ratio of your waist-to-hip measurement is more than 0.8 you can have a greater risk of heart disease, diabetes, osteoporosis and arthritis and you need to take preventative measures.

To calculate your waist-to-hip ratio:

1. Measure your waist at its narrowest.
2. Measure your hips at their widest.
3. Divide your waist measurement by your hip measurement to calculate your ratio.

For example:
79cm (31in) waist divided by 94cm (37in) hip = 0.84

We know that women who are overweight may be more prone to breast cancer because of certain harmful chemicals that can be stored in their body fat – such as xenoestrogens (oestrogen-like chemicals from environmental pollution). Studies have shown that the heaviest 10% of women are 20% more likely to suffer breast cancer than the under-weight 10% at the other end of the weight scale. Fat cells make oestrogen for women of all ages, but as the ovaries decline in their production of oestrogen at the menopause, the body compensates with oestrogen from fat cells.

Apart from problems with heart disease, high blood pressure and diabetes, people who are overweight can have joint pains, arthritis and back trouble because of the excess weight the body is having to carry around.

Fat loss not weight loss

When you say you want to lose weight what you are actually saying is that you want to lose fat. You might assume that as you are losing weight you are only burning off excess fat. If we look at ourselves in simple terms we are made up of fat and lean mass (including muscle). Researchers have found that when women diet, almost 25% of that weight loss can comprise water, bone, muscle and other lean tissue.[7] People on rapid weight loss diets tend to look haggard because they are losing muscle tissue and not much fat. It is physically impossible to lose more than 900g (2lb) of body fat in a week. Real and permanant fat loss has to be gradual and takes time. But it works and the fat stays off.

AVERAGE BODY COMPOSITION OF TYPICAL MEN AND WOMEN

% of body weight	Women	Men
Fat	27	15
Essential fat	12	3
Storage fat	15	12
Bone	12	14.9
Lean tissue	61	70.1
Muscle	36	44.8

The large difference in the essential fat for women includes the fat found in the breasts and in the pelvic area which is necessary for reproduction.

Learn to eat more and lose fat

One of the more surprising but very encouraging facts you will learn from the eating plan in this book is that it is possible to eat more, be healthy and still lose weight. Some foods can naturally actually help us to lose fat – this and other amazing food facts will be explored in later chapters.

CHAPTER 2

Mood, food and cravings

How to banish cravings

There's hardly a dieter in the world who hasn't experienced overwhelming cravings. You can stick quite happily to a diet for days, sometimes for weeks, then suddenly all the good work is blown in one stupid ten minute eating frenzy. It is like having two voices inside your head where one is saying 'you know you don't really need that bar of chocolate' and the other one is saying 'a little bit won't make any difference'. If you listen to the second voice it doesn't stop at a little bit. Before you know it you've eaten the whole bar, maybe even a second. You dread your scale check, you are filled with anger, and having decided that you've ruined that particular day's dieting you might as well make it a complete day of food fun and have chips and syrup pud for dinner. But why? Why do we suddenly go off the rails like that? Is it just greed getting the better of us or is it much more fundamental?

Greed or need?

Occasionally cravings can be put down to greed, but in my opinion it's much more likely that a craving is a biochemical urge that's very, very difficult to control. The body is demanding a particular type of food, usually sugar, because it has a need for it, and when the body has a need it certainly lets us know!

Diet gurus will tell you that the way to banish cravings is to keep all tempting foods out of sight and out of reach. When a craving strikes, they'll suggest you suffer through it, which, as anyone who has experienced cravings knows, is sheer torture! It is also totally non-productive. For as well as anger and guilt, it fosters feelings of self-denial and eventually a dieter can end up feeling useless, worthless and deserving of being fat and ugly.

Rather than banish tempting foods from sight it is better to change your biochemistry so that your body does not have such uncontrollable needs.

Sounds difficult? No, it is so simple that you will wonder why nobody explained it to you before. Cravings are linked with mood swings and if you adjust your biochemistry you will find yourself in control of those cravings. This chapter contains the key to controlling those Jekyll and Hyde mood swings – including pre-menstrual ones – and will help you on your way to successful weight loss.

Blood sugar

Almost all dieters have an underlying blood sugar imbalance. Blood sugar can be the most important factor in losing and maintaining a healthy weight. The importance of correcting blood sugar fluctuations to lose weight is emphasised by the title of an article published in the *Encylopaedia of Common Diseases* written by the staff of *Prevention Magazine*; 'Low Blood Sugar Can Make You Fat'.

Fluctuations in blood sugar can cause:

- cravings
- water retention
- excess thirst
- mood swings

Moods can swing from euphoric to unhappy; angry to couldn't care less; irritable and anxious to bored and tired. The positive moods can be as dangerous as the negative, because you are likely to swing rapidly from one extreme of mood to the other. You must take control of those highs and lows because the associated food cravings can undermine your efforts to change your eating patterns.

Perhaps you know that you are only overcome by cravings for sweet things at pre-menstrual times. If so, this chapter will later explain how blood sugar levels are connected with our hormones.

Nutrition and blood sugar

Nutrition is the key to stabilising the levels of blood sugar. After a meal, glucose from the breakdown of food (digestion) is absorbed through the wall of the intestine into the bloodstream. At this point, there is, quite naturally, a high level of glucose in the blood. The body takes what it immediately needs for energy and then produces insulin from the pancreas in an attempt to lower the level of excess glucose. Any glucose that is not used immediately for energy is changed into glycogen and stored in the liver and muscles to be used later. The glucose level in the blood then reduces to normal.

How do we maintain glucose levels?

To maintain this balance in our blood sugar the body works in a similar way to the thermostat on a central heating system. Our natural 'thermostat' clicks into action as glucose levels rise and fall.

The body takes action in the following ways:

When the glucose level falls too low:
The hormone adrenaline is released from the adrenal glands and glucagon is produced from the pancreas. Glucagon works in the opposite way to insulin and increases blood glucose by encouraging the liver to turn some of its glycogen stores into glucose to give us quick energy. If the blood glucose level stays low for a period of time hypoglycaemia – low blood sugar level – can occur.

Symptoms include: irritability, aggressive outbursts, palpitations, lack of sex drive, crying spells, dizziness, anxiety, confusion, forgetfulness, inability to concentrate, fatigue, insomnia, headaches, muscle cramps, excess sweating and excessive thirst.

Sounds familiar? Chances are that if you have a history of dieting then some or many of those symptoms are known to you. In themselves they can be burdensome, but more importantly they are the outward manifestations that your body is having trouble maintaining a good blood sugar level. They can certainly undermine the efforts of many dieters by triggering unhealthy eating which contributes to weight gain.

When the glucose level rises too high:
Insulin is produced by the pancreas to lower it. If the blood sugar level remains too high, this causes the symptoms of hyperglycaemia – high blood sugar level. The extreme form of this is diabetes which is a medical condition needing expert attention and often entailing regular insulin injections. Weight cycling – weight gain, loss, then gain – may make you more prone to diabetes. Obese people have a 77 times higher chance of developing diabetes than a person at their correct weight – the greater your weight, the higher your risk of developing diabetes.

During a normal day, the amount by which our blood sugar level rises and falls depends on what and when we eat:

What we eat or drink
When we eat any food in refined form its digestion is very fast. Refined foods

have been stripped of their natural goodness by various manufacturing processes. Two of the most widely-used refined foods are sugar and white flour. When digestion is too fast glucose enters the bloodstream too rapidly. This also happens when you take in any food or drink that has a stimulant effect, like tea, coffee, sugar and chocolate. This sharp, fast rise in blood glucose makes you feel momentarily good, but the 'high' quickly passes, plummeting you to a low point, making you feel tired and drained. So what do you need? Another stimulant like a bar of chocolate or cup of coffee (or both!) to give you another boost.

This second boost will cause the blood sugar level to go up rapidly again, and so the vicious cycle is repeated. As blood sugar levels go up and down, so too do our eating patterns, encouraging cravings for sweet foods and drinks.

Over time, this constant over-stimulation exhausts the pancreas. Then, instead of too much insulin, it produces too little. Too much glucose stays in the blood, causing the symptoms of high blood sugar levels.

You are advised to eat natural wholefoods which are unrefined and full of goodness. Their merits in helping to maintain balanced blood sugar levels are discussed later in this chapter.

When we eat or drink

If there is a long gap between eating, the blood glucose will drop to quite a low level and you will feel the need for a quick boost, for instance a cup of tea and a biscuit. At the same time, the adrenal glands will make the liver produce more glucose.

The combination of these two acts causes high levels of glucose in the blood which again calls on the pancreas to over-produce insulin in order to reduce the glucose levels. The vicious cycle starts all over again and the adrenal glands and pancreas become ever more exhausted.

To solve this problem try:

- Grazing – develop a 'grazing' habit in your eating patterns, eating little but often. Leave behind the dieting philosophy of no food between meals.
- Avoid skipped meals – maybe you thought that if you ate less by missing meals you would lose weight but the resultant swings in blood sugar are setting you up to fail. They create a biological urge that must be satisfied and you shouldn't ignore your body's demands even if you were strong enough.

Make it easy for yourself. If you stop what is causing the biological urge then you won't be constantly at war with your own body.

Effects of adrenaline

If blood sugar levels are frequently low and our system is regularly being asked to pump out adrenaline then our health will suffer. Adrenaline is the hormone most of us associate with stress – it is released for 'fight or flight' and its effect is very powerful. If you were threatened in the street, for example, or faced any kind of physical danger your survival mechanisms would instantly step into action with the adrenal glands producing large amounts of adrenaline.

The effects of adrenaline are:

- the heart speeds up
- the arteries tighten to raise blood pressure – hence a 'beating' heart
- the liver releases emergency stores of glucose to give energy
- the digestion stops because it is not necessary for immediate survival
- the clotting ability of the blood is increased in case of injury

This all means that you have been made ready to run faster, fight back and generally react more quickly than normal. Unfortunately, when your blood sugar level drops during the day or night, adrenaline is released automatically and the body experiences all the above sensations except that there is no outside stress to respond to. When this happens repeatedly, you can experience all the health problems outlined under the hypoglycaemia section earlier in this chapter (page 37). It can also contribute to heart disease by increasing the risk of blood clotting and higher blood pressure and the sudden release of glucose for energy can cause extreme fluctuations of sugar levels in the blood.

These fluctuations in blood sugar create an internal stress which the body then has to deal with. It causes an increase in sodium retention resulting in a bloated feeling. The digestive system will not function efficiently and less stomach acid will be produced, which means that more food is stored as it has not been digested sufficiently. The longer food stays in the intestines and remains undigested, the more calories are absorbed. It is therefore important that food is moved quickly out of the intestines, but not so fast that valuable nutrients are not absorbed. Along with all these changes, the body has to call on supplies of vitamins and minerals to deal with this internal stress. If you are continually stressed, the body becomes increasingly nutritionally deficient.

CRAVINGS AND BINGES – WHAT'S THE DIFFERENCE?

Cravings

Most dieters experience cravings to a lesser or greater degree. With some it is for chocolate, with others it is for biscuits and cakes. Certainly it is sweet foods that most people crave although some dieters crave fats – especially cream and hard cheese. Others, who don't usually have a drink problem, can find themselves craving a glass of alcohol. The sugar cravings are caused by the fluctuating blood sugar levels that we've just looked at. The other cravings could be caused by a food allergy or perhaps a yeast problem (see Chapter 5).

By and large you can control your own cravings, even those linked to the hormonal ups and downs of the menstrual cycle. It might be hard at first but by following the rules in this chapter you will find that with the passing of each successful day it will get easier and eventually the cravings will cease.

Bingeing

Bingeing can signal a more serious problem. Giving in to a craving and eating a bar of chocolate or several biscuits is not bingeing. A binge is eating for eating's sake, almost uncontrollably and even when you aren't hungry. Binge-ers have been known to grab at food with their hands rather than waste time with a knife and fork. There is a desperation about binge-ers who often binge in response to an emotional upset. Eating non-stop until you've finished a family-size tub of ice cream, or a complete gateau, for example, is bingeing. So too is eating to the point of being sick. This is a long way from the normal cravings that most dieters experience.

Binge-ers will often feel physically and mentally ill after they've binged and it can be associated with psychological illnesses, like bulimia. Bulimia is characterised by an insatiable desire for food, sometimes with episodes of continuous eating which is followed by purging and depression.

If you know that you binge it is advisable to see your GP.

How can highs and lows be prevented?

There are three good ways:

1. Eat complex carbohydrates regularly
2. Avoid refined foods, especially sugar
3. Reduce foods and drinks that are stimulants

1. Eat complex carbohydrates regularly

There are two types of carbohydrates, complex and simple. To maintain well-balanced blood sugar levels you should eat foods containing complex carbohydrates that give a slow rise in blood sugar and keep a constant level for about three hours. Then eat again and prevent the level from dropping. Spacing food at three-hourly intervals in this way is a proven solution to the battle with cravings.

Dr. Katharina Dalton, a pioneer in the recognition and treatment of pre-menstrual syndrome (PMS), has found that the symptoms of PMS can be relieved by eating regularly. This stops the blood sugar level from dropping and adrenaline from being released. While Dr Dalton's findings have proved invaluable for PMS sufferers serve to confirm the general theory that actually applies to all of us, including men.

Complex carbohydrates give a slow release of energy because it takes time for the digestive tract to break them down into simpler substances that the body can use. Carbohydrates are a large group of foods that include sugars and starches. They are an important source of energy and the body breaks them down into the simple sugar, glucose. It is the slow speed with which this happens that is important to keeping blood sugar constant.

Foods containing simple and complex carbohydrates include:

Complex	*Simple*
Grains (wheat, rye, oats, rice, barley, maize)	Fruit
	Honey
Pulses (lentils, chickpeas, kidney and aduki beans etc.	White and brown sugar
Vegetables, including potatoes	Glucose in high-energy drinks
Fibre in grains, beans and vegetables (see page 42)	

To help maintain a steady blood sugar level, aim to eat complex carbohydrates as part of your main meal and also as snacks during the day. You do not necessarily need to eat great amounts – sometimes just an oat cake can be enough between meals to keep eating urges at bay.

If you find the symptoms associated with low blood sugar level are greatest first thing in the morning, or you wake during the night, heart pounding, and cannot get back to sleep, then it is very likely that your blood sugar level has dropped overnight and adrenaline has kicked into play. Eating a small, starchy snack, like an oatcake, one hour before going to bed and, if possible, one hour after getting up will help to alleviate these symptoms.

Make sure your complex carbohydrates are unrefined, which in general means choosing brown instead of white. For example, wholewheat bread, brown rice and wholemeal flour as opposed to the white versions which have been refined and therefore stripped of essential vitamins, minerals, trace elements and valuable fibre content. In order to digest these refined foods your body has to use its own vitamins and minerals, so depleting your own stores.

Fibre

It was originally thought that fibre's role was only to speed up the passage of food residues to prevent constipation. It is now known that some forms of fibre can actually slow down the absorption of sugars and help to maintain our blood sugar balance. Without fibre, food will affect the blood sugar level more quickly and it is harder to eliminate the food residues. The food stays in the body longer, which means it absorbs more calories so preventing you from shedding those kilos.

Cravings and food allergies

If you experience cravings it's likely to be an indication that you suffer from blood sugar imbalance. They may also be symptoms of a food allergy, so this is worth checking. Ironically, if we are allergic to a particular food, we tend to crave it and eat it more. Ask yourself: 'Which foods or drinks would I find hard to give up?' The answer will give you a clue as to what you could be allergic to. (We will be looking more at allergies in Chapters 5 and 8.)

Shirley had been experiencing bad PMT symptoms and throughout the month would feel extremely hungry by about 5pm even though dinner was not until 6pm. We talked about her pattern of eating and she said that she was drinking up to eight mugs of tea a day. I explained the effects of drinks like tea and coffee on blood sugar balance and their link to PMT symptons and advised her gradually to wean herself off drinks containing caffeine. Unfortunately, Shirley decided to cut out the eight mugs of tea straight away and rang me a couple of days later complaining of a bad headache and flu-like symptoms. Cutting caffeine out of your regime really must be done over a few days and it is best to begin by having half your drinks caffeinated and half de-caffeinated. Then over the next few days reduce the amount of caffeinated cups even further. Eventually you should cut out even de-caffeinated coffee because it still contains stimulants despite the absence of caffeine. Gradually introduce herb, fruit or grain tea so that you are still drinking the same amount of liquid. Once Shirley had taken the advised course of action it took her just a few days to feel a lot better. By the time I saw her two cycles later she was eating little and often and this pattern of eating had really helped with the PMT symptoms.

2. Avoid refined foods, especially sugar

The simple carbohydrates (with the exception of fruit) are all refined foods and should be avoided. Although fruit contains fructose (fruit sugar) which is a simple sugar, the fibre content of the fruit is a complex carbohydrate which slows the digestion rate. So fructose is acceptable when taken in the whole fruit, like an apple, but not when used in the refined form of powdered white fructose, which is bought in boxes.

Pure fruit juice can also cause a rapid change in blood sugar levels because it is not buffered by the fibre that is normally present. It is better to dilute fruit juice in water to make it less concentrated.

Sugar sneaks unexpectedly into many foods. By the way, the brown-is-best theory doesn't apply to sugar: all colours do the same damage to your blood sugar balance! A can of cola may contain up to 120ml (8 teaspoons) of sugar as may a pot of fruit yoghurt. Most of the convenience foods and drinks we buy are laden with sugar including savoury foods such as baked beans and mayonnaise. Did you know that tomato ketchup has just 8% less sugar, weight for weight, than ice cream and that the cream substitute for coffee is 65% sugar compared to 51% for a chocolate bar?

Sugar is an inexpensive bulking agent. Even some toothpastes contain sugar, but as toothpaste is not a food, sugar does have to be included in the ingredients list.

When sugar is in its natural form – the whole sugar cane – it is fine to eat. It has all the right amounts of fibre and is a wholefood. When it is refined sugar is just 'empty' calories – it contains no nutritional value so you can stop eating it and lose nothing but weight.

You may be tempted to substitute sugar with artificial sweeteners – **DON'T!** You are simply introducing an alien chemical which the body then has to deal with. Nobody really knows what havoc these chemicals can cause when introduced to the body's own delicately balanced biochemistry.

If a food or drink is described as 'low sugar' or 'diet' it will usually contain a chemical sweetener. These are also found in some non-diet crisps, ice lollies, sauces, pot noodles and some over-the-counter medicines. It's worth checking labels carefully. If in one day you have several foods and drinks containing artificial sweeteners, there is a cumulative effect by the end of the day. We will be looking at artificial sweeteners and label-reading in Chapter 4.

3. Reduce foods and drinks that are stimulants

Sugar, tobacco, caffeine in tea, coffee, chocolate and caffeinated soft drinks are all stimulants and cause a fast rise in blood sugar level followed by a quick drop which contributes to the roller-coaster ride of blood sugar swings. Avoid them whenever possible even better, cut them out of your diet completely. Substitute them with, for example, herbal teas, grain coffee, spring water and diluted pure fruit juices.

DO

- Eat plenty of unrefined complex carbohydrates including: wholewheat bread, wholemeal pasta, potatoes, brown rice, millet, oats, rye
- Eat fruit and drink diluted pure fruit juice
- Always eat breakfast – porridge oats are good
- Eat small, frequent meals no more than three hours apart if you are a woman or five hours if you are a man (male metabolism is slower)
- Reduce, preferably avoid, stimulants including tea, coffee, chocolate, tobacco and canned drinks that contain caffeine
- Consider taking one of the excellent food supplements on the market that can help balance your blood sugar while you are changing your eating patterns. These are explained in Chapter 7
- Develop the habit of reading labels carefully

DON'T

- Eat refined carbohydrates – avoid 'white' in general. White flour is in many things like cakes, biscuits, pastries and white bread
- Eat sugar or the foods containing it – including chocolate, sweets, biscuits, pastries, soft drinks.
- Substitute decaffeinated coffee (as it contains two other stimulants, even when the caffeine is removed)
- Eat convenience foods as they are likely to contain refined carbohydrates, sugar and high levels of fat and salt

How do you know if your blood sugar is fluctuating?

See how you answer the following questions:

1. Are you rarely wide awake within twenty minutes of rising?
2. Do you need tea, coffee or a cigarette to get you going

in the morning?
3. Do you really like sweet foods?
4. Do you crave bread, cereal, popcorn or pasta?
5. Do you feel you 'need' an alcoholic drink on most days?
6. Are you overweight and unable to shift the extra kilos?
7. Do you often have energy slumps during the day or after meals?
8. Do you often have mood swings or difficulty concentrating?
9. Do you get dizzy or irritable if you go six hours without food?
10. Do you often find you overact to stress?
11. Do you often get irritable, angry or aggressive unexpectedly?
12. Is your energy level less now than it used to be?
13. Do you ever lie about how much sweet food you have eaten?
14. Do you ever keep a supply of sweet food close to hand?
15. Do you feel you could never give up bread?[1]

If you answered 'yes' to eight or more of the questions above, then it is very likely that your blood sugar is fluctuating quite markedly during the day and making you prone to cravings, mood swings and creating difficulties with weight loss.

(The above questions are reproduced with the kind permission of Patrick Holford, author of *The 30 Day Fat Burner Diet*.)

NEW KNOWLEDGE

As more nutritional knowledge becomes available to us through research, more theories circulate about what is good for us and consequently advice changes. Over time we have been told to eat margarine as butter was not good for us, but now scientists realise that the actual process of making margarine produces unhealthy fats (see Chapter 3) and so butter is back in favour.

GLYCAEMIC INDEX

The latest theory in nutrition is the Glycaemic Index which has an important impact on blood sugar balance. As already mentioned, some carbohydrates have a 'fast-releasing' effect while others are 'slow-releasing' and it has been found that this releasing effect can be measured against glucose. This method of measuring has become known as the Glycaemic Index (GI). As glucose is the fastest-releasing carbohydrate, and raises insulin to the highest level, the Index gives it a score of 100 – everything else is measured against this score (see below).

Sugar makes you fat

It is known that raised insulin levels encourage fat to be stored in the body. But if you have high insulin levels because your blood sugar keeps fluctuating, you will not only change more of your food into fat, you will also stop your body breaking down previously stored fat. In effect, it's a bit like adding money to your bank account without spending any: fine with cash but not with fat. No wonder they are called 'fat deposits'!

It is therefore important to put into practice the recommendations mentioned in the first half of this chapter in order to optimise insulin levels and keep fat storage to a minimum. Whole foods, such as brown rice, are important because the fibre contained naturally in the food slows down the release of sugars and gives them a lower GI. The same goes for fruit rather than fruit juice because of the fibre content of the fruit. The most important confirmation that has come out of the Glycaemic Index is that it is beneficial to combine proteins and carbohydrates at the same meal.

The idea of combining protein and carbohydrates makes sense and has been practised for centuries in traditional cultures where a meal would automatically contain foods such as lentils and rice. The Japanese, for example, often have rice, fish and soya at each meal along with vegetables. It was virtually unheard of to see an overweight Japanese person until the introduction of the Western diet in Japan.

The presence of protein in food (either animal or vegetable e.g. tofu) actually lowers its Glycaemic Index. So pulses such as lentils, which naturally contain both protein and carbohydrate, have a low Glycaemic Index.

Food Combining diets (or Not Food Combining as they really are) can be very helpful for people with digestive problems such as indigestion, but can actually make things worse for those with blood sugar imbalance. We are all individuals, so it is important to keep in mind our own circumstances.

THE GLYCAEMIC INDEX OF COMMON FOODS[2]

Sugars	*GI Score*
Glucose	100
Honey	87
Sucrose (sugar)	59
Fruit	
Watermelon	72
Pineapple	66

Melon	65
Raisins	64
Banana	62
Kiwi fruit	52
Grapes	46
Orange juice	46
Apple juice	40
Orange	40
Apple	39
Plum	39
Pear	38
Grapefruit	25
Cherries	25

Grains and Cereals

French baguette	95
White rice	72
Bagel	72
White bread	70
Ryvita	69
Brown rice	66
Muesli	66
Pastry	59
Basmati rice	58
White spaghetti	50
Porridge oats	49
Instant noodles	46
Wholegrain wheat bread	46
Wholemeal spaghetti	42
Wholegrain rye bread	41
Barley	26

Pulses

Baked beans	48
Butter beans	36
Chick peas	36
Blackeye beans	33
Haricot beans	31
Kidney beans	29

Lentils	29
Soya beans	15
Vegetables	
Parsnips (cooked)	97
Potatoes (baked)	85
Potatoes (fried)	75
Potato (boiled new)	70
Beetroot (cooked)	64
Sweetcorn	59
Sweet potatoes	54
Potato crisps	54
Peas	51
Carrots	49

It is interesting that potato crisps have a lower GI than baked potatoes due to the added fat. A woman who came to see me said that she had been feeling drowsy after lunch but after one particular meal, while she was out with a friend, she felt herself falling asleep soon after the food. She had chosen a baked potato with Coronation chicken and salad for lunch. It is possible that the potato was the cause of the problem. If you do feel drowsy after eating, it would be worth keeping a diary for a while to see if you can see a pattern. Do you feel tired when you have a meal that contains foods that have a high GI Index?

It is also fascinating that the GI of wheat will change depending on how it is processed, but the GI of oats stays the same whether they are in the form of porridge oats, oat cakes or oatmeal.

How can the Glycaemic Index work in everyday life?

With glucose given a score of 100, the recommendation is that we eat foods that have a Glycaemic Index of around 50. Foods over 70 should be kept to a minimum or mixed with low GI foods.

However, as fascinating as the GI Index is, it would not be a good idea to swap one one set of restrictive numbers (i.e. calories) for another. You are advised to make yourself aware of those foods that have the highest GIs and eat them in moderation. We should be able to eat everything in moderation and not only stay healthy but also control our weight.

PSYCHOLOGICAL TIPS

What can you do about food cravings?

1. Know your triggers

Become aware of when you crave certain foods. Keep a food diary and identify situations that cause you to overeat. If you know that certain situations make you feel the need for certain foods, either avoid them or prepare yourself by taking something with you to eat that may satisfy that need in a healthy manner.

2. Ask yourself if your emotions are a trigger

Are you eating differently when you feel sad, lonely, stressed or bored? Jane Wardle, a lecturer at London University, found that stress can play a large part in weight control. She sat two groups of people in front of a stressful film and gave them peanuts and Maltesers and observed them. The non-dieters nibbled absent-mindedly but the dieters ate three times the quantity of food. So dieting and stress is a lethal combination.

Look at what else you could substitute instead of food. Fill your life with other things which will keep you active, keep your mind off the subject of food and help keep negative feelings at bay. Find a new hobby, perhaps one you enjoy doing at home, especially in the evenings, like knitting, sewing or reading. Join an evening class – learn to scuba dive! Bring some excitement into your life!

3. Be aware of habit eating

It is very easy to get into habits such as eating while driving or eating while watching television. These can become so ingrained that you can end up always associating food with specific activities. Eating while busily doing something else is a dangerous combination because we become unaware of the quantities we are eating. If the evenings while watching TV are particularly difficult for you, then try doing something with your hands at the same time such as sewing or knitting.

Have a look at what has become automatic. Do you always buy something to eat on the way home from work, or go straight to the fridge when you get in? This action can be almost unconscious. A vital key is to become aware of what you are doing and when. Stop, think and ask yourself: 'Do I really need to eat this now? Will I be happy with the way I feel after I have eaten it?' Ask yourself if you are actually hungry or could you in fact be thirsty? Sometimes these messages get confused, and we are really feeling dehydrated rather than hungry. Try drinking a glass of mineral water, then see if you still feel hungry. Enjoy your food. If you decide to eat a bar of chocolate then just eat the bar of chocolate. Don't watch television or read the newspaper while you do it. Taste the chocolate and eat it slowly, aware of the textures and flavours. Don't feel guilty about eating.

4. Exercise

Exercise releases chemicals called endorphins that make you feel good. Going for a brisk walk or a swim when you feel cravings for food can even ward off the urge to binge. The exercise will also suppress the appetite for a while afterwards. If you tend to eat when you are angry or stressed, try going for a vigorous walk as soon as negative feelings strike.

5. Distract yourself

Cravings will subside even if you don't satisfy them. Do something else, read or make a phone call, and see what you feel like after that.

6. Don't deny yourself

If you say to yourself you are never going to eat chocolate again, you will almost certainly fail. Be realistic. We are all going to eat foods that we are really better off without. If the main foundation of your nutrition is good, relax. Go away on holiday and eat what you like. If you are out with friends for a treat, don't exclude yourself if they are eating ice-cream. If you keep denying yourself you will develop problems of self-denial and the craving may just get to explosion point with you eating far more than if you had allowed yourself a small treat now and again. But this should soon become a problem of the past anyway. If you follow my recommendations, eating little and often with good amounts of complex carbohydrates, you will find your cravings will go automatically without your having to use much willpower. Then you can have a treat without worrying that it may spark off an avalanche!

Mary came to see me with digestive problems and a feeling of being constantly tired. She had a lot of flatulence and felt bloated after each meal, saying it felt as though she was 'eight months pregnant'. She also mentioned having sugar cravings which were 'stronger than those for cigarettes'.

She was put on a supplement programme including chromium (see Chapter 7) and we talked about blood sugar swings and the need to eat little and often with more emphasis on eating complex carbohydrates.

At our next consultation she said that she now 'believed in miracles'. She was sleeping more soundly, her digestion was better and she was eating more regularly. She particularly noticed a difference in her energy levels.

A letter she sent later said: 'I'm happy to report that I have felt very much more energetic. So much so that a couple of people have commented on my jaunty behaviour.'

MOOD AND FOOD

Food and mood are intertwined. There isn't a dieter in the world who doesn't know that to be true. In fact, there's many a weight-watcher who can trace the beginning of their weight problem to a time of emotional turmoil.

Chocolate lovers

When we are depressed we need to cheer ourselves up and what better than with something we love to eat? Be honest: just how often is that 'treat' a chocolate bar? There are substances in chocolate that do indeed impart the 'feel good' factor; in fact they produce the same chemical buzz that we get when we are in love.

In the September 1996 edition of the scientific journal *Nature* researchers showed that the chemicals in chocolate targeted the same brain receptors as marijuana, suggesting that both chocolate and marijuana may share a similar chemistry. Chocolate's effect was definitely milder than marijuana's, but it may explain why chocolate is eaten at times of stress or depression.

Eating for comfort

Scientists have now found that foods can trigger important changes in our brain chemistry. What we eat and drink can determine whether we feel happy or depressed. These powerful brain chemicals can also affect our appetite and our ability to control it. Many of us eat more when we are feeling sad, lonely, depressed, angry, humiliated, belittled, betrayed and other such negative feelings. We eat for comfort and also to ward off boredom. Becoming aware of what controls our appetite and eating patterns is crucial when it comes to losing weight and establishing a healthy way of eating.

Brain chemicals

Within the brain there are chemicals known as neurotransmitters which transmit signals to neurones (brain cells). Some of these brain chemicals control our appetite which is vital for us to survive. We need to feel hungry to keep us alive and yet we also need to feel satisfied to know when to stop eating.

These brain chemicals *increase* our intake of food:

- endorphins
- norepinephrine (noradrenaline)
- neuropeptide Y

These brain chemicals *decrease* our intake of food:

- cholecystokinin (CCK)
- serotonin
- corticotropin releasing factor

How do these brain chemicals make us *feel*?

- Serotonin makes us feel calm and sleepy and can lift depression.
- Norepinephrine (noradrenaline) makes us feel alert and energetic.
- Endorphins can give a 'natural buzz' – a sense of euphoria.

Complex carbohydrates, found in foods such as rice and oats, are said to increase the levels of serotonin which control our appetite and make us feel good. A high-carbohydrate meal causes a larger proportion of tryptophan, an amino acid, to get to the brain to stimulate the production of serotonin.

Carbohydrates help the body to release insulin, and this increases the uptake of the other amino acids, leaving the tryptophan to dominate. On the other hand, when you eat a protein meal or snack, a number of amino acids including tryptophan are competing to get into the brain and therefore the trytophan cannot dominate.

Therefore complex carbohydrates make you feel happier and more relaxed and control your appetite for the next meal. Eating little and often and keeping your blood sugar in balance means that you can control your moods and also your appetite without feeling deprived or hungry. If you eat too little, your serotonin level, which regulates mood and appetite, will fall and then you start to overeat.

Protein contains an amino acid called tyrosine which manufactures the neurotransmitters norepinephrine (noradrenaline) and dopamine which helps to focus our mind and keep us alert.

How can this be applied to everyday life?

Understanding the different biochemical reactions of food on our mood means we can use it to our advantage and eat the right foods at the right time.

For example:

Breakfast – Having a mainly carbohydrate breakfast, such as porridge oats, has a positive mood-enhancing effect. It is important to eat breakfast, but if you find that this makes you feel hungry all day, you should eat a mainly protein breakfast, such as scrambled eggs, with a slice of wholemeal bread.

Lunch – To feel alert and focused in the afternoon, eat a predominantly protein meal for lunch such as a tuna salad with a small portion of rice or Ryvita. If you have a mainly carbohydrate meal, such as a jacket potato, it can make you feel relaxed and sleepy. The body naturally has a 'post-lunch dip' in the afternoon and a carbohydrate meal at lunch will promote this. Many countries enjoy a siesta after lunch but in the UK such a luxury does not fit into the working day and, if affected, we have to battle our way through this afternoon slump. It may be that you crave sweets and chocolates mid afternoon and, if so, you will need to eat a lunch consisting mainly of complex carbohydrates as well as an afternoon snack.

Dinner – If you are turning to alcohol to help you relax in the evening, have a mainly carbohydrate evening meal such as rice and tofu stir-fry.

We are all different. Look at your own daily pattern and work out what different kinds of food are appropriate, and at which times for you.

OTHER WAYS OF CONTROLLING YOUR APPETITE

- Eat more slowly so that your brain, and in turn your appetite, has time to receive the signals that tell it you have eaten enough. The chemical cholecystokinin (CCK) is released as food enters the stomach. It tells the digestion to slow down and then gives the message to the brain that you are 'full' and your appetite naturally decreases. This message takes time – normally about 20 minutes.

- Exercise – interestingly, the neurotransmitter neuropeptide Y is increased when you exercise, stimulating the appetite but making you want to eat complex carbohydrates. These release serotonin which makes you feel good and keeps your appetite under control.
- Eat a wide and varied diet – the balance of the brain chemicals can be disturbed by nutritional deficiencies and by poor diet. The more restricted your choice of foods, the harder it is for your body to help the brain to maintain this important balance of neurotransmitters.

CHAPTER 3

A way of life – not a diet

The best kept secret of weight loss and good health is to eat as naturally as possible. Natural foods are the ones your body can digest easily and use to maximum benefit. These are the foods you can burn off swiftly which means they are good suppliers of energy and don't linger in the body causing weight gain.

To make sure that your daily food intake consists mainly of these types of food is not so much a matter of adopting a diet but more of adopting a new way of life. It's a pattern of eating that will stand you in good stead for the rest of your life. It will still help you to lose weight and keep it off, but the other benefit from eating this way is that it keeps you healthy.

Research by scientists worldwide is now showing that if you look after yourself you have a better chance of preventing certain degenerative illnesses such as heart disease, diabetes and cancer including breast and bowel cancer.

As an analogy, if you put poor-quality petrol into a high-performance car it may run for a while but eventually it will become less efficient and the engine will deteriorate. It is exactly the same with the human body. You need top-grade 'fuel' to 'run on all cylinders'.

Survival is your body's top priority and it will use whatever nourishment you give it to stay alive. Providing it with a quality diet will naturally ease the body's task to keep you healthy and it will also help you maintain a comfortable weight.

The eating plan outlined in this chapter is an enjoyable, pleasurable and healthy way of eating. It won't give you the very quick, early weight loss that accompanies so many diets but you will see a gradual reduction in weight which will be far easier to maintain.

This is not a way of eating to be followed for a short while and then abandoned for former unhealthy eating patterns. The idea is that you embrace a whole new concept of nourishing yourself that is full of variety and very tasty. By eliminating foods that are not good for you and concentrating on foods that are you will find this falls into a pattern that is easy to follow.

There may be occasions when it is not possible to follow the guidelines exactly, perhaps when you are being entertained by others, but so long as you have a foundation of eating well, then the odd deviation from this will not matter.

Above all, food is to be enjoyed. Eating is a time for sharing and socialising. There's nothing more demoralising than turning down invites to eat with friends because you are frightened you will slip from your diet.

Gradually change your eating habits

Some changes to make your eating more healthy are fairly easy to adopt – such as drinking diluted pure fruit juices instead of squash. Others may be harder – such as giving up coffee, tea and sugary snacks. Don't be discouraged because you think that altering your eating habits sounds too difficult. Try taking it one step at a time. You'll be pleasantly surprised at how well you can adapt to changes if you make them gradually. Once you start to feel and see the benefits, you'll know that it was all worthwhile.

This chapter aims to help you make the necessary changes by explaining how different foods and drinks affect the body. Once you understand these effects, you can take control of your weight and health.

It's true – you are what you eat

All the food and drink that goes through your mouth strengthens or weakens, helps or hinders, nourishes or depletes you. Food needn't be your enemy – it's a valuable friend and not something to be fought.

The physiological functions described in this book can be quite technical but are explained here in simple terms:

The body is approximately 63% water, 22% protein, 13% fat and 2% minerals.

Water is an essential nutrient that is involved in every function of the body. It helps transport nutrients and waste products in and out of the cells.

Protein is the basic building block for all your cells and bones plus your hair, skin and nails. It is made from twenty-five amino acids, eight of which are called 'essential' because you must get them from your diet while the other seventeen can be made by your own body. To make sure you are getting the 'essential' eight it is vital to eat protein-rich foods which include eggs, cheese, fish, meat, pulses, nuts and seeds.

Fat is important as it keeps you warm, insulates your nerve cells and is the component of every human cell. Some fats are essential while others aren't we will look at the difference later in this chapter.

Minerals are a natural part of your make-up and are vital for your survival.

The primary source of energy that keeps all this functioning properly and gives you energy for living are carbohydrates which come from grains (rice, wheat, oats, corn, etc.), fruits, vegetables, pulses and beans.

The easiest way to think of your choice of food is to use the food pyramid (below). It was originally developed by the US Department of Agriculture and is now accepted by medical and nutritional experts worldwide. The pyramid divides food into sections, with the ones you need most forming the base and those you need least at the peak.

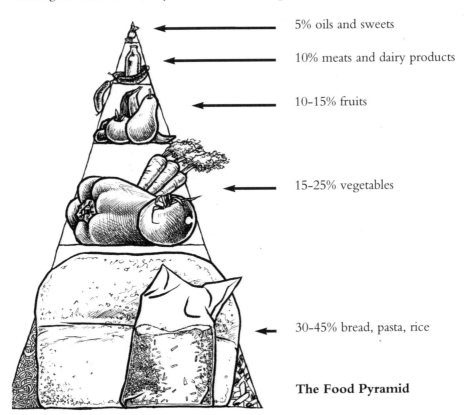

5% oils and sweets

10% meats and dairy products

10-15% fruits

15-25% vegetables

30-45% bread, pasta, rice

The Food Pyramid

This doesn't mean that every single meal should comprise the proportions shown by the pyramid but simply that your eating pattern, say over a week, should be along these lines. If you find a week too long, then think daily. Such a model for eating means that there is no more need to count calories or weigh foods. Freedom at last!

Steps towards a new way of eating

Even accounting for personal preferences and different lifestyles there are certain steps we can *all* take to improve our health and maintain a healthy weight.

1.   Eat regular amounts of complex carbohydrates and fresh fruit.
2.   Stabilise blood sugar levels by reducing your input of refined foods.
3.   Avoid tea, coffee and alcohol – they are not only stimulants but are also addictive. They contribute to the problem of blood sugar level and deprive the body of vital nutrients and trace elements.
4.   Reduce your intake of dairy products and meat.
5.   Ensure your eating plan contains sufficient essential fatty acids and a minimum of non-essential fatty acids.
6.   Check that you are eating enough fibre from natural sources.
7.   Reduce your intake of sodium, which can cause problems with water retention.

Let's now look at each of these areas in more detail:

1. EAT REGULAR AMOUNTS OF COMPLEX CARBOHYDRATES AND FRESH FRUIT

The benefits from eating complex carbohydrates and fruit are discussed in Chapter 2 page 41 – please refer back if you missed it.

2. STABILISE BLOOD SUGAR LEVELS

This is vital to successful weight loss and was discussed in Chapter 2 where we looked at its link to cravings. But even if you don't have a problem with cravings, you still need to stick to the general guidelines to avoid fluctuations in blood sugar levels. So if you skipped that chapter, please go back and read it.

3. Avoid addictive drinks

Alcohol, tea and coffee are socially acceptable drugs and they have an anti-depressant or stimulant effect upon us. Because they are part of everyday life we tend to forget their addictive properties. When we are younger, we are adaptable, flexible and able to eliminate toxins with ease. As we get older our bodies have less tolerance and the effects accumulate. What we could get away with as teenagers we can no longer as we move into our thirties, forties and so on. As our bodies become less efficient we end up storing too much of what they don't actually need.

Coffee

Coffee contains three stimulants – caffeine, theobromine and theophylline. A cup of instant coffee contains around 66mg of caffeine. Freshly ground coffee contains even more. As outlined in Chapter 2, the stimulant effect is often quickly followed by a 'downer' which encourages us to have another cup, and so the cycle is born. The diuretic effect of caffeine may flush vital nutrients and trace elements out of the body. If you are concerned about water retention and are consciously increasing your fluid intake (as you should) don't also increase the amount of coffee you drink. Stick to non-stimulant drinks like water, herbal teas, grain coffees and diluted pure fruit juices. Another problem with coffee is that the active ingredients in caffeine called methylxanthines have been linked to a benign breast disease known as fibrocystic disease. Many women experience breast discomfort in the week before a period that can become worse and develop into mastalgia (which literally means pain in the breast). The pain can be very intense and can occur at any time of the month. By cutting out coffee women have found relief from mastalgia. These methylxanthines are in all caffeine products so chocolate, some canned drinks, cocoa and tea can also be culprits.

Tea

Tea contains both caffeine and tannin. While an average cup of tea contains less caffeine than coffee – about 50mg per cup – the belief that that tea is better for you isn't true. All the above effects of caffeine still apply. As for tannin, if you are a tea-guzzler it not only makes your teeth go brown, it also binds important minerals, preventing their absorption in the digestive tract. If you drink tea, don't have it with a meal because the vital nutrients from that meal will be wasted as they will be excreted unabsorbed.

Are decaffeinated drinks the answer?

Not really. Although decaffeinated coffee does not contain caffeine, it still contains theobromine and theophylline which are two chemicals that can disturb normal sleep patterns. Also they still contain the substances than cause breast problems. Most decaffeinated coffee has been decaffeinated by a chemical which can remain in the product.

Caffeine withdrawal symptoms

Thankfully, more and more people are now becoming aware of the health problems associated with addictive drinks and are turning to alternatives. However, as with all drugs there can be quite dramatic withdrawal symptoms if you stop too suddenly. These include:

- headaches
- nausea
- tiredness
- depression

Some hospitals have now discovered that certain post-operative symptoms are not caused by the effects of the anaesthetic as previously thought, but by caffeine withdrawal. Before a general anaesthetic patients are asked not to eat or drink for a number of hours and by the time they come round from the operation the withdrawal symptoms have already started.

If you have decided to cut caffeine from your diet minimise these possible side effects by cutting down slowly over a period of a few weeks. Gradually substitute some of your usual drinks for more healthy alternatives.

Kate came to see me with a long history of anxiety. For a number of years she had been on and off anti-depressants and felt she was going in a downward spiral with mood swings, depression, dizziness and attacks of paranoia. She was also spotting from mid-cycle until her period arrived. Her GP told her she was depressed and her gynaecologist advised her that her symptons were caused by lack of oestrogen. She wanted to try for a child but said she couldn't imagine ever feeling well enough. I looked at Kate's nutrition which showed that every day she was drinking six cups of tea plus some coffee, and eating four or five biscuits and also cake on top of her regular meals. We talked about the effects of tea and coffee and the possible link between what she was eating and drinking and how she was feeling.

Kate stopped drinking tea and coffee and got headaches for three days while her body adjusted. She also took my advice and changed her eating pattern. Her anxiety and mood swings went completely. What amazed her most was the difference in other aspects of her health too. For the first time in three and a half years she had not spotted before her period came. She had also gone regularly to the toilet each morning, which she hadn't done for ten years as she had been constipated. She feels so much better that she has now decided to try for a baby.

Alcohol

Consumption of alcohol, especially wine, has been rising steadily in the UK. Most alcoholic drink is made by the action of yeast on sugar, so provides calories in the form of carbohydrate. One glass of wine provides us with 100 calories and a pint of beer with around 200 calories. Not only does alcohol contribute to blood sugar imbalance but excessive drinking can also cause liver damage. Furthermore, it acts as an anti-nutrient: i.e. it blocks the good effects of our food by depleting vitamins and minerals, especially zinc. It also interferes with the metabolism of essential fatty acids which are necessary to keep our saturated fats under control and to produce prostaglandins, chemicals that help to control moods and immunity.

What about the 'French paradox'?

The French consume at least the same amount of saturated fat as we do and possibly more, and yet their rate of heart disease is much lower than that in the UK. It was originally thought that wine, especially red wine, was protecting the French from heart problems, but now it seems that the protection is not from the alcohol in the wine but the actual grapes the wine is made of. Grapes produce a substance called resveratrol and in animal studies this has been shown to reduce blood fat and cholesterol levels. So save alcohol for special occasions and eat more grapes!

4. REDUCE YOUR INTAKE OF DAIRY PRODUCTS AND MEAT

Excess protein has been linked to kidney stones, gout and high blood pressure. As we saw from the food pyramid (page 57), a certain amount of protein is essential. It is necessary for the structural formation of our bones, skin, hair and muscle. However, it is important to monitor our intake of protein to ensure that we are not only getting the correct amount but also that it is coming from the healthiest sources.

Red meat which includes beef, pork, lamb and game should, in my opinion, be omitted completely. These have been linked to illnesses such as diverticulitis, a condition in which parts of the colon protrude, forming small pouches which can become inflamed. In 1997 the government's Department of Health Committee on Medical Aspects of Food and Nutrition Policy (COMA) took the rare step of publishing a report entitled *Nutritional Aspects of the Development of Cancer*, which suggested a possible link between the consumption of red meat and bowel cancer. It suggested that intakes at or above the current average of around 90g (3.2oz) per day should be reduced. When you consider that an average portion of bacon is 45g (1.6oz) while just two pork sausages weigh approximately 100g (3.5oz) it makes you realise how easy it is to eat far too much. The Committee's other recommendations included maintaining a healthy body weight, increasing our intake of a wide variety of fruits and vegetables and upping levels of dietary fibre.

An interesting study in 1996 by the Harvard School of Public Health looked at protein consumption and increased bone fractures in women aged between 30 and 55. The researchers found that women who ate more than 95g (3.4oz) of animal protein a day had an increased risk of forearm fractures over women who ate less than 68g (2.4oz) per day. No increased risk was found for those women who ate vegetable rather than animal protein.[1]

Poultry and eggs should be bought with care. Choose free-range eggs which have been produced without the use of growth promoters, antibiotics or hormones. Ensure that all chicken, preferably organic, is thoroughly cooked to kill off any harmful bacteria.

Dairy products such as cheese, milk and cream should be used sparingly as they contain the protein casein. Casein is 300 times higher in cow's milk than it is in human milk, therefore it is hardly surprising that many people find it indigestible. While its casein-richness is important for the fast development of large bones in calves, it can make some people quite unwell. The human digestive system is not designed to receive cow's milk. The cow has a four-stomach digestive system which deals with the casein easily. We humans with our different digestive tract cannot easily absorb the casein, so products like milk remain undigested in the gut and begin to putrefy and rot. It clings as undigested matter to the lining of the intestines and prevents the absorption of vital nutrients by the body. Your body will use much more energy to digest foods that don't suit it. Most people can digest small amounts of milk quite adequately, but if you feel tired after eating it may be worth checking whether your meal contained a lot of milk – perhaps in the form of custard or sauces on vegetables. If your body cannot digest food efficiently it will find it harder to shift the excess weight you have and can even cause you to put on weight.

Dairy produce can sometimes cause problems such as eczema, a runny nose and catarrh.

Nowadays cows are fed antibiotics to speed their growth and hormones to increase their supply of milk. A generation ago an individual cow would produce approximately 9 litres (2 gallons) of milk per day; now it yields 56 litres (12 gallons) per day. The farmers who produce milk from sheep and goats seem to be more ecologically aware and do not interfere with nature to boost the milk yield artificially, so it is better to choose dairy products from these animals.

Yoghurt

Yoghurt is beneficial for health when it contains the culture Lactobacillus acidophilus which is a natural inhabitant of our gut. When, during production, yoghurts are heat treated they lose this original culture so no benefit is gained from eating them. Buy natural yoghurt that is 'live' and organic if possible. This can be marketed in different ways, so read the labels carefully. 'Bio' usually means 'live' and can contain a culture such as lactobacillus acidophilus. Beware fruit yoghurts which can have a very high sugar content. The best yoghurt to choose is natural organic bio yoghurt to which you can add your own fruit.

Recommendations for reducing your intake of red meat and dairy products

Include:

- Fish, poultry, free-range eggs
- Organic goat's, sheep's or cow's milk in moderation. (If you suspect an allergy then go to a good nutritional therapist)

- Live, natural yoghurt with *Lactobacillus acidophilus*
- Nuts, seeds, grains, beans, tofu

Avoid:

- Beef, pork, lamb and game

5. KNOW YOUR FATS

The important point about fats is that some are essential and good for you and some are definitely not. Unfortunately the bad name that fat has gained for itself over the years has unfairly affected the whole family of fats with the result that too many people are trying to stop eating fat altogether.

There are low-fat diets and no-fat diets, both of which can be dangerous. Your body's only source of essential fats is from your diet, so to cut out all fat is not sensible. Indeed fat-free diets have resulted in joint stiffness and skin problems.

When considering fats, it is vital to appreciate the difference between those that can contribute to poor health and those that are necessary for good health. Basically, there are two types – saturated and unsaturated.

Saturated Fats

Saturated fats come from animals (meat, cheese, eggs, etc.) and also from palm kernel oil. These are not essential for your health and in excess they can cause serious health problems. They are detrimental in two ways:

(i) They increase fat deposits
The more saturated a fat becomes, the harder it is to digest and it will be deposited and stored unhealthily in the body. Hence the connection fat intake has with weight gain and narrowing of the arteries. The saturated fat assimilated most easily by the body is butter, followed by coconut oil and palm oil. Fat from beef, lamb and pork are the hardest to digest because they are hard at body temperature.

(ii) They block the use of the essential fats
Saturated fats interfere with your unsaturated fats. Unsaturated fats include the essential fatty acids which, as their name implies, are essential for health.

Unsaturated Fats

It is known that the Eskimos eat large amounts of fat yet have a low rate of heart disease. Why? Because they eat the right sort of fat. The Eskimos' main diet is oily fish which contains essential fatty acids.

Unsaturated fats include essential fats, which are a vital component of every human cell. The body needs them to insulate nerve cells, keep skin and arteries supple, balance hormones and keep you warm. They have also been found to relieve benign breast disease, most especially fibrocystic disease, which is also linked with caffeine intake.

Esential fatty acids are found in nuts, seeds and vegetables. A handful of nuts or a salad dressing made with a good quality oil is sufficient for your daily intake of fatty acid. Also try including in your diet oily fish (such as mackerel or sardines) or take an oily fish supplement.

Unsaturated fats fall into two main groups: monounsaturated and poly-unsaturated.

(i) Monounsaturated fats are so called because chemically speaking they only have one double bond. Olive oil is high in these fats.

(ii) Polyunsaturated fats can have two or more double bonds. Sunflower oil is high in polyunsaturated fat. Within this group there is a further split into Omega 6 fatty acids (the most important of which is linoleic acid) and Omega 3 fatty acids (the most important of which is alpha-linolenic acid).

- *Omega 6* is found in unrefined safflower, corn, sesame and sunflower oils.
- *Omega 3* is found in fish oils and linseed (flax) oil, with varying amounts in pumpkin seeds, walnuts and dark green vegetables. Omega 3 is often lacking in our diet but is very beneficial to health as it has been found to enhance immune function, improve energy levels and soften the skin. Also it increases metabolic rate, so adding Omega 3 to your eating plan can actually help you to lose weight.

  The body makes beneficial prostaglandins (hormone-like regulating substances) from Omega 3. These are particularly useful as they help lower blood pressure, decrease inflammation and decrease sodium and water retention. They also help protect against heart attacks and strokes.[2] A 1986 study published in the *Journal of the National Cancer Institute* showed that linolenic acid killed human cancer cells in tissue culture without harming the normal cells.[3]

Choosing and using oils

Careful choice, storage and use of oils is essential as they can easily be damaged if oxidation takes place. This leaves the oil open to attack by highly reactive chemical fragments called free radicals. It is these free radicals that have been linked to cancer, coronary heart disease, rheumatoid arthritis and premature ageing. Free radicals speed up the ageing process by destroying healthy cells as well as attacking collagen ('cement' that holds cells together) which is the primary organic constituent of bone, cartilage and connective tissue.

As we get older, there is a decrease in collagen, which can cause many changes to the body.

For example:

- skin can become wrinkled
- veins are more prominent
- wounds may heal more slowly
- we bruise more easily
- nails may become brittle
- eyes feel dry and develop dark circles underneath
- gums may bleed or become prone to infection
- hair can look dull with split ends, grow less and maybe even fall out
- bad breath and mouth ulcers develop

Anyone over forty has almost certainly experienced one or more of these but if we avoid free radicals we can reduce the incidence of such problems. Try taking these measures:

Choose cold-pressed unrefined vegetable oils or extra-virgin olive oil

Unfortunately, most supermarket oils are manufactured with chemicals and heat so that the maximum amount of oil is extracted from each batch. This destroys the quality of the oil and its nutritional content. Anti-foaming agents may also have been added to the oils. These excessively processed Omega 6 oils have been linked to enhanced tumour formation.[4]

Avoid hydrogenated vegetable oils

These are listed in the ingredients of most margarines and also many fast foods, crisps, biscuits and crackers. The process of hydrogenation changes the essential unsaturated fats contained in the food into trans fatty acids which have been linked to an increased rate of heart attack.[5] It is for this reason that you are advised to use butter (in moderation), especially organic butter which even supermarkets sell now. Alternatively use unhydrogenated margarine which is available from health food shops.

Why shouldn't I eat the famous-brand vegetable-based margarines?

Although margarine is manufactured from polyunsaturated fats it is made into a solid form through hydrogenation. The process of hydrogenation, explained here, makes terrifying reading:[6]

1. Vegetable oil is mixed with fine particles of nickel or copper.
2. The mixture is heated to approx 200 degrees centigrade for 6 hours.
3. Meanwhile, hydrogen gas is pumped through the mixture at high pressure and the excited hydrogen atoms penetrate the vegetable oil molecules and chemically change them into 'trans fats' (trans fatty acids). These are new, complex substances that are not found in nature, except at low levels in some animal fats. The mixture must be kept very hot – if it cools down at this stage the whole production line will get clogged.
4. Next it is cooled to form tiny hard plastic-like beads, known as hydro-genated oil.
5. These beads are mixed with liquid oil and heated up again to a high temperature. When this cools you have margarine.

Because these trans fats are not natural in such high levels and have a plastic-like quality, your body has great difficulty in trying to eliminate or utilise them. They will be stored then as excess fat if it can't get rid of them. The body is then put under extra pressure to deal with a substance that you do not really need to eat.

Kitchen tips

- Do not fry polyunsaturated fats as they can become oxidised when heated. Use olive oil or butter for frying (monounsaturated olive oil has less chance of creating free radicals while butter never creates them because it is saturated). Reduce temperature to minimise oxidation. Keep all fats to a minimum when frying; try to bake or grill instead.

- Do not store oil in clear bottles on a window sill as light can cause damage. Keep them shut away in a cupboard.

Supplementing essential fatty acids

As you eat these fats, your body makes them more and more complex. The Omega 6 series, linoleic acid, is converted to gamma linolenic acid (GLA) which is also found in evening primrose oil. The Omega 3 series starting with alpha-linolenic acid is converted into eicosapentaenoic acid (EPA) which is also found in fish. There are a number of factors that can stop the conversion of linoleic acid into GLA and that are not beneficial.

As these essential fatty acids are so vital it is advisable to buy them as supplements where the conversion has already taken place, that is as GLA and EPA. This acts as a safeguard just in case your body is not converting them properly itself.

Sources of GLA are:

- evening primrose
- borage
- blackcurrant
- starflower

Whichever supplement you choose, do read the GLA content on the back of the container and aim for a supplement that gives you at least 150mg of GLA per day.

To include EPA aim for a fish-oil supplement. Check the label for one that will give you at least 300 mg of EPA per day.

Recommendations for improving your intake of essential fats

Include:

- Cold pressed, unrefined vegetable oils, such as sesame, sunflower or safflower for salad dressing.

- Extra virgin olive oil for cooking .
- Butter in moderation for spreading or cooking, preferably organic.
- Nuts (almonds, pecans, brazils etc) and seeds (sesame, sunflower, pumpkin, etc.) raw, in salads and in cooking.
- Nut butters in moderation – made without sugar or palm oil.
- Tahini (creamed sesame seeds) for sauces and dressings (available from health food shops).
- Oily fish such as mackerel and sardines.
- Unhydrogenated margarines.

Avoid:

- Commercially produced vegetable oils whose labels do not state that they have been cold-pressed or are extra virgin.
- Heating oils to high temperatures.
- Storing oils in the light, i.e. in glass bottles on a window sill. Keep in a cupboard, even in the fridge.
- Roasting nuts as it destroys the oils.
- Palm oil as it is a saturated fat.
- Hydrogenated margarines, i.e. those made with polyunsaturated vegetable oils which have been hydrogenated. Check the labels.

6. INCREASE YOUR NATURAL FIBRE INTAKE

Fibre in its natural form is helpful in balancing blood sugar levels but it is mainly known for its action on the bowel and the beneficial effects for problems like constipation.

Fibre binds water and increases the bulk of the stools so that they are easier to eliminate from the body. It also prevents the putrefaction of food which can result if food stays in the bowel too long. Putrefying food will ferment, causing a build-up of gas leading to problems of bloating and flatulence.

Fibre also aids digestion, increases your feeling of fullness and removes toxins from the body. By increasing the feeling of being full it helps you to feel more satisfied with what you have eaten and lessens the tendency to overeat.

Other health benefits from eating fibre are a reduction in diseases of the colon (including colon cancer), reduced cholesterol levels and assistance in the detoxification of harmful toxins. Fibre also determines how much oestrogen is stored and how much excreted – soluble fibre binds oestrogen so that it is excreted more efficiently. Chronic constipation has been linked to breast cancer. That's not surprising as toxic waste products that are not eliminated properly can end up stored in the body's fatty tissue, including the breasts.

Fibre and its role in the prevention of breast cancer

The importance of fibre as far as breast cancer is concerned has not been adequately stressed. Women worried about breast cancer are often told to watch their intake of animal fat – which is good general health advice. What is not pointed out is that increasing the amount of fibre (fruit and vegetables) in the diet seems to be more important in prevention of the disease.

Beware bran as a source of fibre

Two English doctors, Denis Burkitt and Hugh Trowell, alerted the world to the health benefits of high-fibre foods in the 1960s. They had spent many years working in Africa where they noticed that Africans had a much lower level of diseases such as colon cancer than Europeans. They linked this to the Africans' very high-fibre diet and the connection between plenty of fibre and better health was made. The Africans' source of fibre had been from grains (not wheat) and fruit. Unfortunately, many people misinterpreted the theory and believed they should add bran to food to increase the fibre content – wheat bran was seen as a convenient source of fibre in the UK because it was readily available and relatively cheap. Bran is a refined food because it is contained in the grains of cereal plants and then stripped away to be sold on its own. It contains phytates which have a binding effect on certain vital nutrients such as iron, zinc, calcium and magnesium, making it less easy for the body to absorb these. Eating bran has led to gastrointestinal problems such as irritable bowel syndrome. It makes much more sense to eat the bran in the form that nature intended by eating the grains in their whole state.

Recommendations for increasing natural fibre in your diet

Include:

- Plenty of fresh fruit and vegetables, cooked or raw.

- Whole grains like brown rice, wholemeal bread, wholegrain crackers and brown pasta.
- Pulses in salads or in cooking (tinned for convenience are okay but avoid those with added sugar).
- Nuts and seeds – either raw or in cooking.
- Muesli – soak it first if it contains raw flakes of various grains for at least 10 minutes (but overnight is best). Soaking enables the phytates to be broken down so they do not affect your mineral metabolism.

Avoid or reduce:

- Refined carbohydrates including cakes, bread and biscuits and everything containing white flour and sugar.
- Bran on its own or in breakfast cereals.

Constipation

So what can you use instead of bran if you need help? It is important that your bowels are working properly because their function is to get rid of everything that your body doesn't need. If you are not eliminating toxins and poisons efficiently they can be reabsorbed into your system and cause ill health.

To begin with increase your intake of fresh fruit and vegetables: this should make quite a difference fairly quickly. If you still need more help then either sprinkle 15ml (1 tablespoon) of linseeds on to your breakfast cereal in the morning or soak 15ml (1 tablespoon) of linseeds in a small amount of water and then swallow. Vitamin C can also be used to help soften stools. Try taking a supplement of 1000mg per day and increase by 500mg at a time until your stools are manageable, soft and comfortable.

7. REDUCE YOUR SODIUM INTAKE

Sodium is a mineral that is closely connected with the body's ability to balance water retention and blood pressure. The higher the level of blood sodium, the higher the blood pressure. Another mineral, potassium, works with sodium to regulate water balance and normalise heart rhythm. The more sodium we consume, the more potassium we need to counteract this effect. So we need to do two things: reduce our loss of potassium and reduce our intake of sodium.

1. **Potassium loss** can be caused by low blood sugar, diuretics and laxatives – so avoid all three. Also reduce alcohol, coffee and sugar – all of which make us lose potassium.
2. **Sodium reduction** can be effectively achieved by reducing our intake of salt. Sodium chloride (table salt) is a major source of sodium in the body. It is found naturally in all fruits, vegetables and grains and is already present in most of our ready-prepared foods, including ketchup, salad dressings, burgers, chips, biscuits, pizzas; so we do not need to add more during cooking or at the table.

The World Health Organisation recommends a maximum of 6g (1 rounded teaspoon) of salt a day. This supplies us with 2400mg of sodium. We only need 500mg of sodium a day to keep us healthy. Most people end up eating 9g of salt a day and it is easy to consume too much without realising it. One burger in a bun can contain 6g, two slices of wholemeal bread 1.2g and a slice of cheese and tomato pizza 5.3g. Two slices of bread contain more salt than a packet of crisps. Always read food lables carefully to check for the presence of salt.

We also consume sodium as sodium nitrate which is the preservative used in meat and as monosodium glutamate, the flavour enhancer, used extensively in convenience and Chinese food. Food which is advertised as low fat or low sugar is usually extremely high in salt.

A 1998 Government report on nutrition and heart disease by the Committee on Medical Aspects concluded that the reduction of salt in the diet by a third could save at least 34,000 lives a year.

Also, if we have a high salt intake we can be carrying around an extra 1.8kg (4lb) in weight due to water retention.

Recommendations to reduce sodium intake:

Include:

- More freshly prepared foods so that you are aware of all the ingredients.
- Low-salt alternatives such as Lo-Salt.
- Herbs, garlic, ginger, lemon juice, tamari (wheat-free soy sauce) and miso in cooking to add flavour.
- Read labels carefully.

Avoid or reduce:

- Your use of salt, added at the table or in cooking. If you really must use a little choose sea salt which is free of the chemicals which are added to table salt to make it flow freely.
- Convenience or prepared foods with a high salt content – the food should not contain 0.5g or more of sodium (1.25g salt) per 100g.

Soya

The role of soya in preventing and treating chronic disease has become internationally recognised. When buying soya look out for the natural, non-tampered-with beans.[7] A lot of soya has been genetically modified and this should be avoided – more about this subject later in this chapter.

Soya contains more protein than milk without the saturated fat or cholesterol. Soya beans are the only ones considered to be a complete protein because they contain all eight essential amino acids. They are also high in essential fatty acids and soya milk is naturally cholesterol-free.

Japanese women have minimal menopausal problems; they do not even have a word for 'hot flushes'. They also have one sixth the rate of breast cancer deaths that we have in the West. Studies in the USA have shown that when Japanese women move to the West and adopt a western diet, they develop more cases of breast cancer.[8]

Soya is being studied extensively around the world for its effectiveness in lowering cholesterol and preventing cardiovascular disease, menopausal symptoms and osteoporosis.

In women, body fat is a manufacturing plant for oestrogen, so when you are overweight your oestrogen levels will be higher than normal. You can become slightly heavier at the menopause because this extra oestrogen from the fat cells balances the oestrogen decline from the ovaries. However, being very overweight brings with it excess oestrogen levels which for some women may mean increased risk of breast and womb cancers of which many are oestrogen-dependent tumours. Other conditions which are affected by oestrogen levels include endometriosis, fibroids, heavy and/or long periods and fibrocystic breast disease (lumpy and tender breasts).

Oestrogen is not one hormone but several grouped together, including oestradiol, oestrone and oestriol. It is the liver's job to convert oestradiol (which is the carcinogenic oestrogen) into oestrone and then into oestriol which is non-carcinogenic. It is important that your liver is working efficiently and tips to improve liver function are included in Chapter 7.

How does soya help prevent breast cancer?

Soya is classed as a phyto-oestrogen which means that it contains substances that have a hormone-like action. Soya beans, for instance, contain phyto-chemicals known as isoflavones which make up about 75% of the soya bean protein. Two of the isoflavones in soya are genistein and daidzein. In the human gut, bacteria convert isoflavones into compounds that have an oestro-genic action, although they are not hormones. These phyto-oestrogens seem to fit into oestrogen receptors in the breast but are probably too weak to stim-ulate the cells. What seems to happen is that these weak oestrogens block the oestrogen receptors and prevent cancer developing.[9] In simple terms, they prevent the carcinogenic oestradiol in the body from latching on.

Soya beans have been found to contain at least five compounds believed to inhibit cancer. One of these is chemically similar to the drug Tamoxifen, which is now used to treat oestrogen-dependent breast cancer. Tamoxifen works as an oestrogen receptor antagonist: that is it binds on to the oestrogen receptors and inhibits cancer growth. The Japanese diet includes a large con-sumption of soya bean products including tofu, miso (soya bean paste), tamari (wheat-free soya sauce), tempeh and soya milk. Tests show that the Japanese have high levels of isoflavones in their urine and plasma, indicating that their traditional soya-high diet supplies them naturally with the phytochemicals (plant chemicals) that may prevent hormonally linked cancers. Japanese women have been shown to excrete phyto-oestrogens in their urine 100–1,000 times higher than those excreted by American women.[10]

Soya and its effect on cholesterol

Studies have shown that eating soya decreases the LDL cholesterol ('bad' cho-lesterol) and also the triglycerides.[11] It has also been found that the higher the person's initial cholesterol level, the greater is the effect of the soya. It is esti-mated that taking 25mg of soya protein a day can have this beneficial effect on cholesterol (tofu contains approximately 12g of soya protein per 100g) Two glasses of soya milk provide about 20mg of soya protein, so it is not an excessive amount to eat. How the soya protein has this effect on cholesterol is not yet known but a number of theories have been put forward.

Excretion of bile – It is thought that soya increases faecal excretion of bile acids and by doing this 'pulls' cholesterol from the body.

Thyroid effect – Some studies have found that soya protein increases thyroxine and in some cases thyroid stimulating hormone, which is very relevant in terms of weight loss and boosting metabolism.[12]

Fibre effect – Soya is a soluble fibre which will bind with some of the cholesterol and fat in the food you eat. As the fibre passes out unabsorbed, this also keeps fat levels under control.

Soya and the menopause

There are numerous research papers on the beneficial effects of soya on both reducing hot flushes[13] and preventing osteoporosis.[14] In one study just the addition of 45g of soya flour reduced the number of hot flushes by 40%.[15] With osteoporosis, genistein, one of the soya isoflavones, has been shown to inhibit osteoclasts (which renew old bone by dissolving or reabsorbing it) and stimulating the osteoblasts (cells which replace the old bone with new.[14, 16])

Soya and men

Its logical to ask what the effect on men might be as soya is a phyto-oestrogen. Of course, in Japan both men and women eat good quantities of soya each day. Each year, an increasing number of men in the UK are being diagnosed with prostate cancer and it kills four times more men than cancer of the cervix kills women. Japanese men have the same rate of prostate cancer as men in the UK but they have a lower death rate from this cancer. Japanese men who ate tofu more than five times a week had half the risk of dying from prostate cancer compared with Japanese men who only ate tofu less than once a week.[17] It seems that the phyto-oestrogens in soya can have a balancing effect on hormones in both men and women – without them excess oestrogen in men can trigger the overproduction of testosterone which is a factor in the development of prostate cancer.

GENETICALLY MODIFIED FOOD

Soya is probably the most well known among genetically modified foods and up to 60% of processed foods contain soya including bread, biscuits, pizza and baby food. Lecithin contained in many foods is also made from soya. Just what proportion of that 60% is now genetically modified we do not know, but it is thought to be quite considerable. Apparently the beneficial substances in soya, the isoflavones, are unaffected by the genetic engineering process – but to be on the safe side you are advised to buy the non genetically modified soya.

Other genetically modified foods on sale in the UK are maize, tomato paste and cheese containing chymosin, a genetically modified rennet which hardens the cheese.

Genetically modified foods have been produced by introducing genes from other species to crops to make them more resistant to pests, viruses or weed killers. For instance, it is now possible to buy a tomato which contains a fish gene to boost its frost resistance. As Prince Charles once said: 'Genetic modification takes mankind into realms that belongs to God, and to God alone.'

Even the scientists disagree as to the value and dangers of genetically modifying foods. Dr George Wald, 1967 Nobel Laureate in Medicine, wrote in his book, *The Recombinant DNA Debate*:[18]

> Up to now, living organisms have evolved very slowly and new forms have had plenty of time to settle in. Now whole proteins will be transported over night into wholly new associations, with consequences no one can foretell either for the host organisms or their neighbours . . . going ahead in this direction may not only be unwise but dangerous. Potentially it could breed new animal and plant disease, new sources of cancer, novel epidemics.

Professor Richard Lacey who accurately predicted years ago the problems with BSE has also spoken out against genetically modifying foods.

Dr Mae-Wan Ho, who is a reader in Biology at the Open University, has called for a five year moratorium on genetic engineering. She believes that 'agricultural biotechnology is inherently unsustainable and hazardous to biodiversity, human and animal health... If you mess up life by scrambling the genes then there is no return.'[19]

From September 1998, it has been mandatory to label products containing genetically modified DNA. This labelling only applies to genetically modified soya and maize (corn) products and only where protein or DNA can be detected in the final product by laboratory screening. Foods containing soya oil, refined starches and additives such as emulsifiers and lecithins will be excluded. Greenpeace estimates this means 90% of foods containing genetically modified products will be unlabelled.

Some organisations are making a stand against these so-called 'Frankenstein' foods. The Vegetarian Society has announced that from August 1999 all foods bearing the V symbol will have to be free from genetically modified products. Provamel, the market leader of soya products in the UK, have stated that their foods are free from genetically modified products and have implemented a system of tracing the soya from seed to final production.

The gene manipulation that we are now tinkering with bypasses evolution. As yet we don't know what the price of that tinkering will be. In order to smuggle these new genes across the species barrier, scientists use infectious viruses and bacteria. We could be sitting on yet another health time bomb. One would think the scientists would have learned by now that we cannot manipulate nature without consequences. We know that by feeding cattle-remains to herbivorous cows, the scientists effectively went directly against nature and turned the cows into cannibals.

Another worry is that newly-created genes may escape into the environment and affect other plants and wildlife. As plants are now being developed to tolerate certain herbicides, the intention is that only the weeds will be killed when the crop is sprayed. But could those herbicide-tolerant genes escape to the weeds themselves, making them resistant to the sprays as well? If that happened, ever stronger herbicides would have to be developed. And what would that do to our rivers, our air, our wildlife, our planet? One case of these 'superweeds' has already been identified, where genetically modified resistant genes from oilseed rape (a brassica) crept into wild brassicas. Tests on beneficial ladybirds have found a premature death rate of 50% and a drastic reduction in fertility in cases where the ladybirds had eaten greenfly which fed on genetically modified potatoes.

The argument supporting genetically modifying foods is that we have used biological processes successfully for centuries to improve food supplies. This is true, but these processes did not manipulate genes, which is a more dangerous concept. My advice is to avoid genetically modified foods. If we as consumers consciously do not buy these foods, then eventually there may not be a market for them.

CHAPTER 4

Shop and cook wisely

The key to shopping wisely is to buy your food in its most natural state. Ask yourself what has happened to the food or drink before it reaches the shops? Try to buy organic produce that has not been sprayed with chemicals. Pesticides, DDT and Kepone contain xenoestrogens which are oestrogen-like compounds that can upset the delicate male and female hormone balance. Although DDT is banned in the UK it is still used in some developing countries and can therefore enter our food chain through imported goods.

Become a label detective

If ever there were labels that mattered it's the ones on the food we eat. Yet it seems that we give them little attention. Most of us lead busy lives with little time to spare for reading the small print on food labels. However, it is worth investing some of your time on this important subject. For what we eat can cause problems to our health, not to mention its effect on our weight. Once you begin reading labels you could be in for a big surprise – you probably had no idea you were putting so many chemicals into your system. Initially it will take some time to get used to phraseology and brand differences. You may even find it useful to make notes that you can refer to at any time. But once you are familiar with the best brands to buy, shopping for the healthiest foods will become quick and automatic.

What to look for when checking a food label

The ingredients on a label are listed with the first ingredient having the greatest quantity and the last having the least quantity in that product. Unfortunately, most labels do not tell us exactly how much of each ingredient is in the food; so one fish pie could contain more fish than another and we wouldn't know.

It is best to avoid ingredients which sound like a chemistry lesson. For example, these are the contents of a brand of apricot dessert: sugar, hydrogenated vegetable oil, gelling agents (E331, E401, E431), emulsifiers (E447, E322), adipic acid, lactose, caseinate, whey powder, flavourings, artificial sweetener (sodium saccharin), colours (E110, E122, E102, E160a). So we immediately know that the ingredient with the greatest quantity in this dessert is sugar. But have you spotted something even more important? Where are the apricots? Our commonsense should tell us that this isn't a very natural food.

E numbers

As a general guide avoid products with E numbers. Some are fine to eat, as they are naturally-derived, but the vast majority are not and have known side effects. There are books on the market that provide E-number references which, if you are very diligent, you could carry with you when shopping – but that could make a difficult problem even more wearisome. The best action is to simply avoid Es.

E numbers include permitted colourings (some natural, some not), preservatives, permitted antioxidants (some natural, e.g. ascorbic acid – vitamin C – others not) emulsifiers and stabilisers, sweeteners, solvents, mineral hydrocarbons and modified starches. Some products might list natural annatto colouring on the label, for instance. This is in fact E160b and has no known adverse side effects. If the additive in question is a natural one, many food manufactures now make this clear because it is a good selling point.

E numbers that are okay include:
E100 and 101 riboblavin (VB2); E140; E160A alpha-, beta- and gamma-carotene; E160B, annatto; 160C, E-F; E161, 161A, C-G; E162 (extract of beetroot); E163; E170, chalk; E172; E260; E262-3; E301-9; E322, lecithin; E331 A-C; E335; E337; E400-2; E404-5; E440A-B.

Artificial sweeteners

These are chemicals and the safety of many of them is in doubt so they are best avoided. The US Centre for Science in the Public Interest called for a ban on the sweetener acesulfame-K because it is believed to be carcinogenic.

Chemical sweeteners are used in a wide variety of foods and drinks because, for the manufacturers, they have the advantage of being cheaper than sugar and, in some cases, sweeter. Saccharin, for instance, is 300 times sweeter than sugar. The danger of these sweeteners is not only their individual effects but also the chemical cocktail that results in the body when you consume a number of sweetners from different products.

The artificial sweeteners we are likely to encounter in processed no-sugar and low-sugar foods and drinks or in special diet dishes are described briefly below.

Acesulfame-K: made with sulphur and nitrogen. It was developed in 1967. It is about 200 times sweeter than sugar and is used in soft drinks, preserves, yoghurts, canned foods and confectionery.

Aspartame: made from two amino acids. Often sold under the brand names NutraSweet and Canderel. First discovered in 1965, it is about 180 times sweeter than sugar and is used in soft drinks, yoghurts, chewing gum, ice cream, salads, alcoholic drinks, hot drink mixes and dry mix desserts.

Saccharin: made from petroleum materials. Discovered in 1937, it is about 300 times sweeter than sucrose. Used in soft drinks, canned foods, salad dressings, ice lollies, confectionery and pharmaceuticals including over the counter drugs.

Thaumatin: made from ketemfe, an African plant, and developed in 1968. It is about 2,000 times sweeter than sugar and is found in chewing gum.

The American Cancer Society found that people who regularly use artificial sweeteners tend to gain weight, not lose it and this is because the sweeteners can slow down the digestive process and increase appetite.

Be wary of labels which say 'no added sugar' as it can mean no added sugar of any kind, or simply no added sucrose. Don't assume that the sugar content is very low because a food bears a 'no added sugar' label. In order to make sugar content appear less, some manufacturers break down the sugars into various forms on the label, although they all have relatively the same effects on our bodies.

Words ending in –ose are sugars:

- Sucrose – common table sugar, made from sugar cane or beet
- Fructose – fruit sugar
- Glucose – body blood sugar, fast acting
- Dextrose – sugar from corn starch, chemically identical to glucose
- Lactose – milk sugar
- Maltose – sugar made from starch

Always take into account the total of the sugar figures provided. Be careful too of foods whose labels claim to have 'less added sugar'. For example, a label may say the food contains 25% less added sugar and salt. Although there may well be a reduction the product as a whole could have only 15% less total sugar and 10% less total salt than the original brand.

Hydrogenated vegetable oils

Often found in margarine, crisps, burgers and biscuits, these should be avoided. Look for similar products with 'hydrogenated vegetable oils' in the list of ingredients.

Whey

Whey is the yellow-green by-product of cheese production and should also be avoided. It has a vile taste and an awful smell but is concealed in various food products such as cartoned fresh soup and margarines. Because of the increase in cheese consumption more whey is being produced than ever before.

An article in the *Los Angeles Times*, 4 December 1978, stated:

Not only is there more whey, but it is harder to dispose of. Stricter federal and state regulations prohibit dumping raw whey down sewers. Whey is 100 to 200 times stronger a pollutant than residential sewage and most municipal sewerage plants cannot treat it adequately. Disposal in streams is out because whey depletes waterways of oxygen, rendering them incapable of supporting marine life. Even disposal on used land or gravel pits is often unsuitable because of seepage into water supplies. The solution hit upon by both industry and government is to apply high technology and sophisticated marketing techniques and feed the stuff to humans.

Whey is increasingly showing up as a cheap substitute ingredient in a wide range of processed foods, from bakery goods and ice cream to soup mixes and beverages.

LOOK FOR THE SHORTEST INGREDIENTS LIST

Generally, the longer the ingredients list, the more suspicious you should be about the naturalness of the product. Manufacturers argue that additives, preservatives and flavourings, etc., are used in such small quantities that they will not have any adverse effect. However, when you take into account all the small amounts in all the different products we eat and drink every day, these small amounts soon add up. We are also producing a chemical cocktail inside ourselves and nobody knows how these chemicals will react together.

It is quite impossible to make sure that every single thing you eat is chemical free, especially if your lifestyle means you have to take snacks or meals away from home, as most of us do. Just make sure that what you eat at home is as natural and healthy as possible – 'everything in moderation' is the best rule to follow. If your busy life means that sometimes you have to buy convenience or packaged food, then find the best brand you can and go for the shortest, least chemical-looking ingredients list.

TIPS FOR FOOD PREPARATION AND COOKING

- Organic carrots, potatoes, parsnips, swedes, etc only need scrubbing. Do not peel them as most the nutrients are concentrated just under the skin.
- Lightly cook vegetables in a little water or steam.
- Avoid frying where possible. Try grilling or baking.
- Choose cookware with care. Avoid aluminium as this is a heavy toxic metal that can enter food through the cooking. The same applies to aluminium foil and cases. The best cookware materials are cast iron, enamel, glass and stainless steel.

SHOPPING LIST

Variety is the key to enjoying your food and eating for health and weight control. There may be foods mentioned below that you have never tried, so experiment and enjoy yourself. Many foods are available in supermarkets, others can be bought from good health food shops, wholefood stores or farm shops.

Here is a shopping list for foods that will help you keep your weight under control:

Fruit

Include plenty of fresh fruit, organic if possible. Many supermarkets sell seasonal organic fruit and some health food stores even sell a frozen organic range. It can be slightly more expensive but in health terms is well worth the extra cost. It also tastes better. If you live in a rural area hunt down a local organic farm shop or look out for organic delivery firms. If you have the time you could consider growing some fruits yourself – apart from the fact that they make your garden look delightful you also know for sure that your produce is pesticide free.

Make sure you eat a wide variety of fruits

As well as the usual:
apples, pears, grapes, oranges and bananas.
Remember:
plums, peaches, nectarines, berries, cherries, dates, melons, kiwis, tangerines and satsumas.
For a tropical taste try:
mango, pawpaw, lychee and passion fruit.

Fruit is very versatile. It can be put into pies, tarts and crumbles or just plain stewed. It can be enjoyed raw or mashed into natural live yoghurt and is ideal for any time of the day. If you need to snack away from home it's easy to carry and is good for children's lunch boxes.

Dried fruits

Raisins, apricots, dates, sultanas, prunes, figs, apple rings, etc., make an enjoyable change but eat them in moderation. When buying avoid any that contain the preserving agent sulphur dioxide which is also used as a bleaching agent in flour. Sulphur dioxide occurs naturally but is produced chemically for commercial use. It is suspected of being a factor in genetic mutations and an irritant of the alimentary food canal. Sulphur dioxide is used most often on dried apricots to keep them a 'nice' orange colour. The packet will state whether or not they are free from sulphur dioxide. Those that are free from preservative will look brown but taste fine. Figs and dates are usually free from sulphur dioxide.

Supermarket dried fruits such as mixed fruit, raisins, sultanas, etc., will often have mineral oil added to them. This gives them a shiny appearance and keeps them separate. Try to avoid these as the oil can interfere with the absorption of calcium and phosphorus. As it passes through the body mineral oil can pick up and excrete the oil-soluble vitamins (A, D, E, K) which we really want to retain.

Vegetables and salads

Buy organic if you can and as already mentioned just scrub the skins, don't peel them as you'll lose valuable nutrients which are close to the skin. *All* vegetables are allowed on this eating plan, even the root vegetables like potatoes and parsnips which you've probably tried to avoid in the past as 'fattening'.

You can also enjoy:
artichokes, asparagus, avocado, beetroot, broccoli, brussel sprouts,cabbage, carrots, cauliflower, celeriac, celery, corn on the cob, cucumber, garlic, green beans, kale, lettuce, mange tout, mushrooms, onions, peas, peppers, pumpkins, radishes, runner beans, sugar-snap peas, squash, swedes, sweet potatoes, turnips, watercress, yams.

This list is not complete but serves to show that in the vegetable and salad world everything is good for you.

ENTER THE WORLD OF SEED SPROUTING

Not only are seed sprouts healthy, but they can also be fun. Various seeds and small beans, such as alfalfa, mung beans and chickpeas, will sprout if kept damp in a warm place. Once sprouted they are an excellent source of 'live' nutrition and good to mix in salads.

You can buy them already sprouted from health food shops but you can also sprout them yourself. Health food shops sell special trays which aren't expensive and can be the start of a whole new eating pattern. Keep them, once sprouted, in a polythene bag in the fridge. Rinse the tray and start the next batch. Kids love to watch them sprout.

Grains

If your budget limits the amount of organic produce you can buy, put grains at the top of the shopping list. Grains are very small so will absorb more pesticides than other foods, so it is best to buy organic. You will have no trouble buying organic grains at health food shops if your local supermarket doesn't sell them.

Include:
barley, bulgur, brown basmati rice, buckwheat, cous cous, millet, popcorn (you will need a heavy saucepan for the popcorn), oats (whole jumbo flakes and porridge), long grain brown rice, short grain brown rice

Breakfast cereals

From the supermarket:
Shredded Wheat and Puffed Wheat are sugar-free (as are supermarket own brands of these).

From health food shops:
Suma's Malted Wheat Flakes (just wheat and malt)
Kallo's Puffed Rice Cereal (only organically grown wholegrain brown rice)
Doves' Organic Corn Flakes (organic corn, organic wheat syrup, organic barley malt extract, sea salt)
Silbury's Organic Cereal Crisps (organic rice, organic maize, organic corn malt syrup).

Muesli

There are a number of good mueslis made by Jordans and Country Life and some supermarkets also have their own brands. Muesli contains raw flakes of various grains and must be soaked for a minimum of ten minutes before eating, but soaking overnight is definitely best. Soaking enables the phytates, which can block the uptake of minerals from food, to be broken down properly. If you suspect you have a problem with wheat, you can buy a wheat-free muesli.

Bread

Again, organic is best and choose wholegrain loaves. Wholemeal bread from Doves and Shipton Mill is good. You may also find good bread in your health food shop. A lot of supermarket bread contains either sucrose or dextrose and/or flour improvers, so read the labels. If the flour improver is ascorbic acid that's OK as it is a form of Vitamin C but any other flour improvers are not OK.

Many supermarkets now carry a range of speciality breads such as olive, tomato and pitta. They all make a change but do check the labels for additives. Organic wheat and rye breads are available too. Look out for Manna organic sprouted breads – fruit, multigrain and fruity malt loaf. Rye and pumpernickel breads are also good.

Bread is allowed in your eating plan **BUT** eat it in moderation.

Corn tortilla shells

These are very useful for stuffing with a kidney bean filling. Either soak and cook your own kidney beans or buy tinned. Check the label as some have sugar and salt added.

Crackers and savoury biscuits

There is a wide variety of wholemeal crackers and biscuits available at supermarkets and health food shops. You can also buy organic. Make sure you always read labels carefully for excessive salt content. Ryvita and Wasa are good, as are Kallo organic rice cakes, oat cakes and Doves Farm organic rye biscuits.

Flour

If you are a home baker you will find there are wholemeal organic flours for bread and pastry making. Doves' organic wholemeal pastry flour for cakes and pastries is very good as it is fine milled and very light. Also, supermarkets now sell a good selection of organic wholemeal and unbleached white flours. It is also possible to buy organic self-raising flour.

Pasta

There are a number of brands of wholewheat pastas such as Lima and Record. For a change try the supermarkets' fresh pastas. They are usually made from white flour, but if the rest of your diet is good then it is fine to use these white pastas occasionally.

Supermarkets also sell rice noodles which are excellent in stir fries. Health food shops sell corn and vegetable pastas and buckwheat noodles, all of which are nutritionally good.

Flavourings

Choose from:
ginger, garlic, fresh and dried herbs, lemon juice, sea salt, Lo-salt, miso (soya bean paste, which you can add to cooked dishes or even drink stirred into hot water), mustard (check for added sugar, chemicals, etc.), arrowroot or kuzu for thickening gravies and sauces.

Whole Earth makes a good organic tomato ketchup; Kite makes a sugar-free mayonnaise; and there are a number of ready-made salad dressings with no sugar or chemicals, but do check labels. Cardini's, Newman's and Chalice have good ingredients and are sold in most supermarkets.

Soy sauce

Soy sauce isn't just for Chinese foods, it's good on rice, in salad dressings and sauces. Choose organic where possible and avoid any makes with mono-sodium glutamate. Good brands are Clearspring, Westbrae and Eden.

Nuts

You can enjoy:
almonds, Brazil nuts, cashews, cob nuts, pecans, pine kernels (pignolas), pistachios and walnuts.

Nuts can be eaten as a snack with raisins during the day or used in cooking or salads. Pine nuts added to brown rice during cooking make a healthy and enjoyable change.

Seeds

Try:
sunflower, sesame, pumpkin, poppy and caraway.

Organic are available. They can be added to salads or cooked vegetable dishes or put in with rice when cooking.

Seed and nut butters

Regard these as a treat and eat in moderation.
Try:
Tahini (creamed sesame seeds) – this can be used in salad dressings and is also used in making hummous (the Greek dip made from chickpeas). Sunita makes a no-salt tahini.
Nut butters – Meridian and Whole Earth have a good selection. Try to avoid those that include palm oil, as it is a saturated fat.

Sweeteners

It is better to rely on the natural sweetness of foods themselves than to use artificial sweeteners. If you are making cakes, try adding carrots, raisins or bananas to sweeten them. For apple pies use eating apples so that you do not need to add sugar – you could always add raisins or sultanas to make a pie sweeter. Date slice is wonderful because dates are naturally sweet. As your taste buds grow accustomed to doing without the very powerful taste of refined sugar you will come to appreciate the natural sweetness of vegetables and fruits.

Try using the following as sweetners:
maple syrup, concentrated apple juice, barley malt, date syrup and honey.

You should actually use honey sparingly and avoid types which are 'blended' or the 'produce of more than one country' because they are often heated to temperatures as high as 71 degrees C (160 degrees F) which destroys their natural goodness.

Beware maple syrup labelled as 'flavoured' because it could contain sugar and chemical flavouring. Flapjacks made with barley malt are delicious: try them for a healthy change.

Pulses/legumes

With the help of good cookery books and advice from health food shops, you will soon find that pulses are easy to cook with and very versatile. As with anything new it is just a case of getting used to it.

Try experimenting with:
aduki beans, black-eyed peas, chickpeas (used in hummous), haricot beans (used in baked beans), kidney beans, lentils (brown and red – wonderful for soups, vegetarian shepherd's pie and vegetarian spaghetti bolognese), lima beans, mung beans (known as beansprouts when sprouted), navy beans, soya beans (also used for making tofu, soya sauce and miso), split peas.

Most pulses (not lentils) need to be soaked, some overnight, before cooking. Alternatively you can buy them in tins, but watch labels for added sugar and salt. Pulses make a good base for many healthy dishes, especially if you are trying to cut out meat from your eating plan – they are great added to salads, soups and casseroles.

Meat

Meat contains saturated fat so should be kept to a minimum. Organic meat is better for you as growth hormones, antibiotics and other chemicals are given to many animals reared non-organically for human consumption. Of all meat, poultry is the healthiest choice and you will find several supermarkets now sell organic, free range or corn fed birds. Some meat suppliers will home-deliver organic meat and they are worth looking out for.

A further reason for reducing the amount of red meat you eat is the possible link between the consumption of red meat and bowel cancer. The Government has suggested that the intake of red meat should be less than 90g (3.2oz) a day.

Fish

All fish is good for you. Its saturated fat levels are low and it is very nutritious. Avoid frying – grill or poach instead. Plaice, trout and Dover sole are all good cooked this way. Oily fish is particularly good as it contains high levels of essential fatty acids, so enjoy mackerel, tuna, salmon (eat the bones), sardines and anchovies. Fresh fish is best but frozen or tinned is okay.

Eggs

Buy free-range and preferably organic eggs which will be labelled with words to the effect: 'from hens fed on food free from antibiotics, hormones and artificial growth promoters'. Free-range only implies that the hens, unlike their battery cousins, have been given a degree of freedom. This often means they are kept in huge barns with only a tiny door to the outside – very few are able to reach this door and venture outside. They can also still be fed on 'junk'.

Soya

The value of soya has been discussed in Chapter 3 and it is useful to have on your shopping list. It is a very versatile natural vegetable protein and if you have trouble digesting animal milk or find that it causes skin problems or sinus trouble, soya milk is a helpful alternative.

Soya milk

Buy organic where possible and make sure the milk is sugar-free. Provamel makes an organic sugar-free soya milk – just filtered water and organic soya beans. The Japanese soya milks are also good – one of these is Bonsoy which contains purified water, organic soya beans, barley malt, barley and kombu (a sea vegetable). The Japanese milks do not have the after taste of some soya milks. Soya milk can be used in cooking in the same way as you would use cow's milk – you will find you cannot taste the difference between the two.

Tofu

Soya can also be bought in the form of tofu which is soya bean curd made by adding a curdling agent to soya milk. Tofu can be eaten raw, used in stir-fries, soups and also desserts.

Miso

This is another product made from soya beans which are combined with rice or barley. A mould culture is added and the mixture is left to ferment for one to three years. Miso is bought in paste form and can be added to soups or casseroles. You can also buy ready-made packets of miso soup containing dried tofu – all you need to add is water.

To add miso to your own soup, in a small bowl combine a small quantity of the soup with the miso to make a smooth paste. Heat the soup and, when it is almost ready, add the paste. Once the miso has been added, the heat should be kept very low otherwise the beneficial enzymes in the miso could be destroyed. Only simmer for a few minutes and serve.

When you are accustomed to the flavour, it makes a nourishing drink: just add 5ml (1 teaspoon) of the paste to a cup of boiling water.

Soy sauce (shoyu)

This soya product has already been mentioned as a flavouring. It is made from fermented soya beans and is sometimes sold as tamari which is a wheat-free version. Whichever soy sauce you choose make sure it contains just the natural ingredients: soya beans, wheat, water and salt -not sugar or monosodium glutamate (MSG).

Tempeh

Tempeh is another soya bean product made from fermenting beans pressed into a block. It has a strong taste and can be fried or used in soups.

Dairy produce

Use organic dairy produce where possible. If you have difficulty assimilating cow's milk try sheep's or goat's milk, or a non-animal drink like soya or rice as described above. Buy 'live' or 'bio' yoghurt containing the culture *Lactobacillus acidophilus*. If you like fruit yoghurt then add your own fruit to natural live yoghurt. Frozen yoghurt makes a refreshing summer dessert – use a standard recipe and substitute sugar with maple syrup or honey.

Oil/fat

Use butter, organic if possible, and unhydrogenated margarines. Vitaquell, Vitasieg, both unhydrogenated, can be obtained from health food shops. When buying oils look for cold pressed, unrefined vegetable oils like sesame, sunflower, safflower. Buy extra virgin olive oil for such things as stir fries. Use non-hydrogenated margarines for cakes and pastry.

Rice drinks

Other alternatives to animal milk are rice drinks. They can be used in cooking, on cereals and as a drink, either hot or cold. Good brands include Lima's Rice Drink (water, organic rice, organic safflower oil, sea salt and vanilla) and Imagine Foods' Rice Dream (filtered water, organically grown brown rice, safflower oil and sea salt). These and other brands are available from health food shops and some supermarkets.

Oat drinks

Oat milk is another alternative to cow's milk and is made from a mixture of oats, oil and water. One brand to look for is Mill Milk.

Tea and coffee substitutes

As a substitute for coffee try:
Caro and Caro Extra, Bambu or Yannoh. These are all grain 'coffees' and contain various combinations of ingredients like barley, rye, chicory and acorns.

Instead of tea try:
herb and fruit 'teas', Rooibos which is a South African caffeine-free 'tea' made from a bush of the same name, decaffeinated tea and Japanese bancha (twig) 'tea'.

If you really must have a 'proper' cup of tea every now and again buy organic, available from supermarkets and healthfood shops. Good makes include Ridgways and Clipper.

Herb teas

When you use herb (not fruit) teas on a regular basis remember that herbs have specific effects so it is better to use a variety of herbs rather than stick to one favourite flavour. For example, peppermint is very good for aiding digestion and is good to drink after a meal. Chamomile is relaxing and is often drunk at the end of the day to help insomnia. It also has an anti-inflammatory action which is useful in the digestive system for diverticulitis as well as general colon problems. Reputable manufacturers of herbal and fruit teas include Celestial Seasonings, London Herb and Spice, Heath and Heather, Secret Garden and Dr Stuart's.

Soft drinks

Use pure unsweetened fruit juice. If a carton or bottle has 'fruit drink' on the label then you know that something else has been added. It has been found that many fruit drinks have only 5% fruit, the other 95% being water, sugar and additives. You should be careful about the flavoured spring waters as many contain a surprising amount of sugar. Liven up fruit juice with sparkling mineral water or try the sparkling apple juices, Appletize and Kiri. Aqua Libra and Ame are also good soft drinks. Free Drinks makes a range of sugar-free sodas and Whole Earth makes a wonderful 'real' lemonade and orange soda which are free from sugar, preservatives and artificial colours and flavours. Meridian makes a very good range of concentrated juices in an interesting mix of flavours including apple and blackcurrant, pear, apple and cherry, apple and raspberry. Their apple and strawberry juice is particularly delicious diluted in hot water. All of these are available from health food shops.

Water

Let's not forget this very simple, natural drink. Our bodies are made up of approximately 70% water and this is involved in every bodily process including digestion, absorption, circulation and excretion. We can survive without food for about five weeks but we can't live without water for longer than five days. Water is essential for carrying waste out of the body; it helps with constipation and helps maintain body temperature.

Drink more water

Most of us do not drink enough water and, ironically, people who suffer from water retention tend to restrict their liquid intake thinking the less they drink, the less their bodies will retain. Actually, the opposite is true. If we restrict fluids the body tries to compensate, just as it adopts a famine-mode when food is restricted, and will retain liquid in case it is in short supply. Ideally we should try to drink around six glasses of water a day which should substitute other less healthy drinks. An excellent start to the day is a cup of hot water and a slice of lemon: it's wonderfully refreshing and excellent for the liver.

Which water is best – tap, filtered or bottled?

Tap water can be contaminated with any number of impurities which vary from area to area. Arsenic, lead and copper can all occur naturally in the water and some water can be contaminated by the pipes carrying it. Other substances such as agricultural pesticides and fertilisers can leach into the water through the ground.

Filter water won't eliminate every single impurity but will help. You can buy a jug filter from health food shops, supermarkets, chemists and some ironmongers. Tap water is poured through a cartridge which 'cleanses' the water, but it must be changed regularly or bacteria can flourish. Alternatively, you can have a filter plumbed into your water system before the water gets to the taps – under the sink is an ideal place. Cartridges also need changing with this system. Once you have your supply of filtered water you can use it not only for drinking but also for washing fruit and vegetables and cooking.

Bottled water comes in many guises so here is a short guide to help you understand what you are buying:

- **Spring water** – may have been taken from one or more underground sources and have undergone a range of treatments, such as filtration and blending
- **Natural mineral water** – bottled in its natural underground state and untreated in any way. It has to come from an officially registered source, conform to purity standards and carry details of its source and mineral analysis on the label.
- **Naturally sparkling water** – natural water from its underground source with enough natural carbon dioxide to make it bubbly.
- **Sparkling (carbonated) water** – has had carbon dioxide added during bottling, the same as with ordinary fizzy drinks.

Convenience foods

Baked beans

Be careful with supermarket brands which often contain a fair amount of sugar. If the label states 'sugar-free', the beans may well contain an artificial sweetener instead, so do check the ingredients list carefully. Whole Earth makes excellent sugar-free, organic baked beans which are sweetened with apple juice.

Soups

Again it is difficult to find those which do not contain sugar, artificial sweeteners or chemicals. Baxters have a good range of acceptable soups, including Mediterranean Tomato, Minestrone and Carrot and Butterbean but do check the ingredients before buying. There are now also a number of good fresh soups in the supermarkets.

Ready-prepared meals

Despite your good intentions to eat well it may sometimes be necessary to use ready-prepared food. You should look for the more wholesome types such as Whole Earth and Meridian Italiano sauces which are useful served with pasta when time is really short. Most of the pasta sauces in the supermarkets contain sugar, so keep checking labels until you are familiar with the brands which are best for you. There are some reasonable frozen meals available, but keep these for emergencies as it is best to cook from fresh whenever possible.

Snacks and biscuits

Fresh fruit, dried fruit, nuts and raisins are all good and tasty to use as a snack at any time. You can get good quality crisps and tortilla (corn) chips from health food shops and some supermarkets. Some manufacturers use sea salt in these products. With crisps and corn chips check whether the oil used is non-hydrogenated. Ryvita and rice cakes (there are many flavours) are fine to eat; also oat cakes so long as they do not contain sugar.

There are many sugar-free biscuits available, mainly from health food shops, but supermarkets may sell a few. If you suffer from bloating or digestive problems, you may have a wheat allergy and biscuits and bread will make the condition worse. If you suspect you have this type of problem you should be checked by a good nutritional therapist (see Chapter 7).

Clearspring makes a good range of cookies (sesame, muesli and hazelnut varieties) which contain a high proportion of organic ingredients and are sweetened with maple syrup and corn malt. Infinity Foods sells delicious organic biscuits including carob, carob chip, fruit and nut, malt syrup waffles and hazelnut waffles. Again some of the ingredients are organic and the waffles, for example, are sweetened with maize malt syrup. These would have to be obtained from a good health food shop or you may have to order them.

There are a number of fruit and carob bars on the market which may satisfy your taste for a snack. Never substitute ordinary sweet foods with diabetic ones as these contain sorbitol. This is a sugar alcohol which occurs naturally in some fruits and is metabolised in our bodies. For commercial use, it is synthesised chemically from glucose.

Diabetics are recommended to eat only a certain amount of sorbitol per day because it can have adverse side effects such as flatulence, diarrhoea and bloating. It is also high in calories and can take the place of other more nutritious food. It does not raise the blood-sugar level significantly, as would sugar or pure glucose, but it is not a natural food and should be avoided.

Jams

There are some very good quality sugar-free jams available including Meridian, Whole Earth and some supermarket own-brands. If you see a supermarket jam marked 'sugar-free' check the label for artificial sweeteners. Jam should be made solely from fruit.

There are also some excellent marmalades including St. Dalfour's which is available in supermarkets. Meridian and Whole Earth also have a range of organic jams.

Some jam companies have been known to extract the colour from the fruit during the jam making process and then add artificial colours to give their products a rich colour. Natural jams may not look quite as bright but they are delicious.

Jam spreads are also tasty and should not be overlooked. Officially the word 'jam' means preserve, which implies that it contains sugar to act as a preservative, therefore the natural sugar-free jams have to be called spreads. They contain only real fruit and a natural setting agent such as pectin from limes. The choice of flavours is quite amazing, including apricot, mixed berry, blackcurrant, kiwi, pineapple, plum, morello cherry, peach and passion, blackberry and apple, wild blueberry, wild hedgerow and the usual strawberry and raspberry. Because they contain no preservatives they must be kept in the fridge after opening.

There is also another kind of fruit spread from Suma called 'Pear and Apple Spread' which contains the concentrated juice of pears and apples.

Because it is so concentrated it lasts for months unrefrigerated. It is very dark and thick, quite unlike ordinary jam but well worth trying as it is delicious and different.

Desserts

As you steer away from pre-packaged foods, it becomes more necessary to make your own desserts. For speed and convenience you can eat fresh fruit either whole or cut up as a fruit salad or mixed into 'live' yoghurt. Baked eating apples are easy to prepare with a stuffing of sultanas. Stewed fruit or compotes can also be prepared easily – remember to avoid adding sugar. You'll be amazed at how quickly your taste buds will adapt to less sugar in your food.

Provamel produces a soya carob dessert which is sugar free and Plamil makes a tinned rice pudding with sultanas. Supermarkets have a good range of tinned fruit which is packed in fruit juice rather than syrup. Fresh fruit is always preferable but tinned fruit could be added to a fresh fruit salad for variety.

Seaweed/sea vegetable

The name seaweed is rather off-putting and so I prefer to use the term sea vegetable, which is what it is. Sea vegetables are sold dried in packets in health food shops.

They are low in calories, fat free and are an excellent source of iodine, which is essential to the healthy function of the thyroid gland (which regulates our metabolism). They have a good mineral content including potassium, calcium and copper as well as the trace minerals zinc, manganese, chromium, selenium and cobalt and the macro minerals calcium, magnesium, iron and iodine.

Good seaweeds to try are:
dulse, kombu (Japanese form of kelp), wakame, agar, nori, arame and hiziki.

Sea vegetables can be used in a number of different ways: for example, in soups, salads and savoury dishes (see the recipes in Chapter 9).

A valid criticism of eating sea vegetables is that because they are harvested from the sea they could be laden with pollutants such as lead, cadmium and mercury. However, if you buy from a reputable company such as Clearspring, you can be assured that the sea vegetables are grown in clear water away from known areas of pollution. After harvesting, the sea vegetables are also tested independently for heavy metal contamination.

CHAPTER 5

Still can't lose weight?

If you eat correctly, take proper exercise and yet your weight still does not shift, what do you do? First check with your GP that you do not have a medical condition, such as an underactive thyroid, which is causing the weight gain.

Do you have an underactive thyroid?

If you answer 'yes' to four or more of the following questions then your thyroid could be underactive to some degree and you should visit your GP for a check-up.

- Has your weight gone up gradually over months for no apparent reason?
- Do you often feel cold?
- Are you constipated?
- Are you depressed, forgetful or confused?
- Are you losing hair or is it drier than it used to be?
- Is your skin drier than it used to be?
- Are you having menstrual problems?
- Are you having difficulty falling pregnant?
- Have you noticed a lack of energy?
- Are you getting headaches?

The thyroid gland situated in your neck, together with the hypothalamus and pituitary glands in your brain, helps control your metabolism. It produces two hormones, thyroxine and triiodothyronine, production of which is triggered by the hypothalamus and the pituitary which also produce thyroid-stimulating hormones (TSH) and thyrotrophin-releasing hormones. These hormones are stored in the thyroid until needed. An underactive thyroid, or hypothyroidism, is a deficiency of thyroid hormone caused either by failure of the pituitary gland to produce TSH or failure of the thyroid itself.

It is estimated that there are over one hundred symptoms of thyroid imbalance and, because of this huge range, it often causes confusion in diagnosis. The symptoms can mimic other problems so it may take a GP some time to sort out the real trouble and prescribe the correct treatment. However, there is a blood test available to assess thyroid function and, if you think you have a problem, you should ask your doctor for this test.

Unfortunately mild forms of underactivity go undetected by the test so your GP may not offer medication to assist you. From his point of view the test has shown that your general health is not at risk, which is his prime concern, but it still does not cancel the possibility that a mild thyroid underactivity isn't affecting your weight.

However, before you despair, there is another way to test your thyroid function.

The most popular way of testing thyroid function, before the advent of the blood test, was to measure the basal body temperature. Even if you haven't considered that your thyroid might be underactive it would be worth doing this test at home.

Basal means the body's temperature at rest. If the temperature is too low it may indicate that you have a sluggish metabolism caused by an underactive thyroid.

The temperature is taken once a day for three days. Women should do this test on the second, third and fourth days of the menstrual cycle. The female body temperature rises after ovulation so it would not give a clear picture if done later in the cycle. Non-menstruating women, and men, should take their temperature on any three consecutive days. Basal body temperature should read between 36.4 and 36.7 degrees C (97.6 and 98.2 degrees F).

How to measure your basal body temperature:

1. First get a thermometer. (The traditional type is fine but there are some good electronic ones on the market which only take a minute to register the temperature and bleep when it is done).
2. Put the thermometer by your bed before you go to sleep.
3. On waking remain lying still in bed – do not have a drink or walk to the bathroom before you take your temperature. Put the thermometer in your armpit and leave it there until it bleeps. If you are using

the traditional type leave it for ten minutes, having made sure the mercury was at its lowest point before you began.
4. Make a note of your temperature on each of the three mornings and calculate your average temperature.

If your average temperature falls below 36.4 degrees C (97.6 degrees F) then your thyroid may not be functioning properly. It would be well worth giving your GP these results and asking for the blood test. If you have already had the GP's blood test and he was happy that there was nothing amiss with your thyroid, but your home test shows a low basal body temperature, by all means speak to him again. Alternatively consult a good natural medicine practitioner who will be able to prescribe non-drug remedies.

Metabolic rate

Your metabolism is the total of all the calorie-burning changes that occur in the body. These changes are fuelled by the energy converted from food you eat and trigger essential physiological functions such as cell renewal, digestion, hormone release and brain activity. Laboratory tests can gauge how many calories you need to burn daily but few of us have access to such facilities.

Your resting metabolic rate (RMR) is the amount of calories you burn every day simply by being alive. The RMR is expressed as calories because it is a measure of the amount of heat liberated during the metabolic process. Exercise, body temperature, hormone changes and digestion can all increase metabolic rate. You can estimate your own RMR with a simple calculation:

1. If you are under 31 multiply your weight by 14.7 and then add 496.
2. If you are over 31, multiply your weight by 8.7 and then add 829.

(Note: For this you will need to input your weight in kilograms – divide pounds by 2.2 to convert to kilograms)

Any extra calories you may need depend on your activity level so:
- If you are sedentary multiply your RMR by 1.4.
- If you are moderately active (mostly seated during the day but take some exercise) then multiply your RMR by 1.7.
- If you are very active during the day and take organised exercise more than four times a week then multiply your RMR by 2.

Metabolism and exercise

An inactive woman of about 1.68m (5ft 6in) and weighing 60kg (9.5 stone) will have a resting metabolic rate of 1,400 calories whereas if she exercises regularly then she will probably burn off about 2,400 calories a day. It's virtually impossible for this woman to gain weight, indeed if she goes on doing this day after day she will lose a lot of weight. It just proves how important exercise is to weight control (see Chapter 6). If the same woman was eating 3,000 calories a day she would slowly gain weight and would therefore need to exercise more.

Metabolism and digestion

Our metabolic rate increases during digestion of food; this is called the thermal effect of food. This is why it is important to eat little and often. Even after just five hours without food the body starts to believe it is being starved and will decrease its metabolism. So after seven or eight hours of sleep and then missing breakfast, you are putting your body into fasting mode and you are more likely to store fat rather than use it.

Ideal weight

How do you know what your ideal weight is? According to the height and weight tables everybody of the same height is expected to weigh the same – but of course they don't. Although people may be of the same height they can have quite different body shapes – some may have big hips, some big breasts, some small feet. Also, fit people will often look slim but can weigh more because of an increased muscle mass, and it is even possible to be underweight but have a high percentage of fat. Thin people can still have cellulite because of the storage of fat on the thighs.

Set point weight

There is a weight that your body is naturally drawn to which is called your set point weight. If you eat well and healthily with a good level of physical activity then your body will automatically reach this weight. Many people diet for years and when they eventually get down to a certain weight they can't lose any more. Very often this is their ideal weight but they continue to force themselves to try to lose more. The only way to do that is by starvation and then, of course, when they start to eat normally again the weight rushes back on. It is this acceptance of our own constitution, our own genetic make-up that is the key ultimately to our health and happiness. On any street we would expect to see a wide range of heights in people and we accept this as normal so we should also accept that there is a wide range of body shapes and sizes. There are some women who are a size 8 and no matter what they eat they do not gain weight: that is their constitution.

BODY MASS INDEX

If you want to have a rough idea of your 'ideal' weight then the Body Mass Index (BMI) is the best indicator. It tries to identity the percentage of body tissue which is actually fat. There are disadvantages with this measurement because it does not allow for variations in fat, bone, organs and muscles. So a fat and a thin person who are the same weight and height can have the same BMI. Equally a fit athlete and a couch potato can have the same BMI because lean muscle weighs more than fat.

Some fitness centres use pincer-like tweezers (called skinfold calipers) to measure percentage of body fat. The thickness of the skinfold can give an indication of the amount of fat stored under the skin. At least three different places on the body need to be measured and a chart gives the estimate of body fat from the sum of the three sites. There are also electronic machines which use bioelectrical impedance: an electric current is passed through the body and the machine measures how long it takes for the current to come out, giving an individual's total body fat. Lean tissue is a much better conductor of electricity than fatty tissue so the machine can measure the percentage of fat in the body.

Your BMI is a ratio of height to weight and is calculated as follows:
BMI= your weight in kg divided by the square of your height in metres. For example, if your weight is 63.5kg (10 stone) and your height is 1.68m (5ft 6in), your BMI = 63.5 divided by (1.68 x 1.68) = 22.5.

If your BMI is 20-25 you are normal weight; 25-30 indicates you are overweight; 30-40 indicates you are obese; 40 plus indicates you are dangerously obese.

A BMI of around 30 would indicate a woman of average height being around 15.8kg (2½ stone) overweight.

stn's	kgs \ ft	4.8	4.9	4.10	4.11	5.0	5.1	5.2	5.3	5.4	5.5	5.6	5.7	5.8	5.9	5.10	5.11	6
	cms	142	145	147	150	152	155	158	160	163	165	168	170	173	175	178	180	183
6.4	40	20	19	19	18	17	17	16	16	15	15	14	14	13	13	13	12	12
6.6	41	20	20	19	18	18	17	16	16	15	15	15	14	14	13	13	13	12
6.9	42	21	20	19	19	18	17	17	16	16	15	15	15	14	14	13	13	13
6.11	43	21	20	20	19	19	18	17	17	16	16	15	15	14	14	14	13	13
6.13	44	22	21	20	20	19	18	18	17	17	16	16	15	15	14	14	14	13
7.1	45	22	21	21	20	19	19	18	18	17	17	16	16	15	15	14	14	13
7.3	46	23	22	21	20	20	19	18	18	17	17	16	16	15	15	15	14	14
7.6	47	23	22	22	21	20	20	19	18	18	17	17	16	16	15	15	15	14
7.8	48	24	23	22	21	21	20	19	19	18	18	17	17	16	16	15	15	14
7.10	49	24	23	23	22	21	20	20	19	18	18	17	17	16	16	15	15	15
7.12	50	25	24	23	22	22	21	20	20	19	18	18	17	17	16	16	15	15
8	51	25	24	24	23	22	21	20	20	19	19	18	18	17	17	16	16	15
8.3	52	26	25	24	23	23	22	21	20	20	19	18	18	17	17	16	16	16
8.5	53	26	25	25	24	23	22	21	21	20	19	19	18	18	17	17	16	16
8.7	54	27	26	25	24	23	22	22	21	20	20	19	19	18	18	17	17	16
8.9	55	27	26	25	24	24	23	22	21	21	20	19	19	18	18	17	17	16
8.11	56	28	27	26	25	24	23	22	22	21	21	20	19	19	18	18	17	17
9	57	28	27	26	25	25	24	23	22	21	21	20	20	19	19	18	18	17
9.2	58	29	28	27	26	25	24	23	23	22	21	21	20	19	19	18	18	17
9.4	59	29	28	27	26	26	25	24	23	22	22	21	20	20	19	19	18	18
9.6	60	30	29	28	27	26	25	24	23	23	22	21	21	20	20	19	19	18
9.9	61	30	29	28	27	26	25	24	24	23	22	22	21	20	20	19	19	18
9.11	62	31	29	29	28	27	26	25	24	23	23	22	21	21	20	20	19	19
9.13	63	31	30	29	28	27	26	25	25	24	23	22	22	21	21	20	19	19
10.1	64	32	30	30	28	28	27	26	25	24	24	23	22	21	21	20	20	19
10.3	65	32	31	30	29	28	27	26	25	24	24	23	22	22	21	21	20	19
10.6	66	33	31	31	29	29	27	26	26	25	24	23	23	22	22	21	20	20
10.8	67	33	32	31	30	29	28	27	26	25	25	24	23	22	22	21	21	20
10.10	68	34	32	31	30	29	28	27	27	26	25	24	24	23	22	21	21	20
10.12	69	34	33	32	31	30	29	28	27	26	25	24	24	23	23	22	21	21
11	70	35	33	32	31	30	29	28	27	26	26	25	24	23	23	22	22	21
11.3	71	35	34	33	32	31	30	28	28	27	26	25	25	24	23	22	22	21
11.5	72	36	34	33	32	31	30	29	28	27	26	26	25	24	24	23	22	21
11.7	73	36	35	34	32	32	30	29	29	27	27	26	25	24	24	23	22	22
11.9	74	37	35	34	33	32	31	30	29	28	27	26	26	25	24	23	23	22
11.11	75	37	36	35	33	32	31	30	29	28	28	27	26	25	24	23	23	22
12	76	38	36	35	34	33	32	30	30	29	28	27	26	25	25	24	23	23
12.2	77	38	37	36	34	33	32	31	30	29	28	27	27	26	25	24	24	23
12.4	78	39	37	36	35	34	32	31	30	29	29	28	27	26	25	25	24	23
12.6	79	39	38	37	35	34	33	32	31	30	29	28	27	26	26	25	24	24
12.8	80	40	38	37	36	35	33	32	31	30	29	28	28	27	26	25	25	24
12.11	81	40	39	37	36	35	34	32	32	30	30	29	28	27	26	26	25	24
12.13	82	41	39	38	36	35	34	33	32	31	30	29	28	27	27	26	25	24
13.1	83	41	39	38	37	36	35	33	32	31	30	29	29	28	27	26	26	25
13.3	84	42	40	39	37	36	35	34	33	32	31	30	29	28	27	27	26	25
13.5	85	42	40	39	38	37	35	34	33	32	31	30	29	28	28	27	26	25
13.8	86	43	41	40	38	37	36	34	34	32	32	30	30	29	28	27	27	26
13.10	87	43	41	40	39	38	36	35	34	33	32	31	30	29	28	27	27	26
13.12	88	44	42	41	39	38	37	35	34	33	32	31	30	29	29	28	27	26
14	89	44	42	41	40	39	37	36	35	33	33	32	31	30	29	28	27	27
14.2	90	45	43	42	40	39	37	36	35	34	33	32	31	30	29	28	28	27
	cms	142	145	147	150	152	155	158	160	163	165	168	170	173	175	178	180	183
	ft	4.8	4.9	4.10	4.11	5.0	5.1	5.2	5.3	5.4	5.5	5.6	5.7	5.8	5.9	5.10	5.11	6

Use this chart to find your Body Mass Index Imperial measures given are only approximates.   BMI = kg/m^2

Another way to calculate ideal weight is described in *Columbia's University College of Physicians and Surgeons Complete Home Medical Guide* (1985):

1. Divide your height in inches by 66.
2. Multiply the answer by itself.
3. Multiply the result by 100 and then add your age.

The answer from this total (in lb) is the middle of the range. Within 7–8lb either side of this ideal weight is still healthy for most people.

Brown fat and yellow fat

We *need* body fat. It insulates us from the cold and keeps our skin and arteries supple. There are two kinds of fat cells, brown and yellow (sometimes called white). Brown fat is darker as it contains a large number of mitochondria (power houses) which are portions of cells where energy is made and burned off. Because brown fat has a large number of mitochondria it means it is very metabolically active and a great deal of energy is burned. Yellow fat is not so active and it is this fat that tends to accumulate in various parts of the body, especially on women, and especially around the hips, abdomen, thighs and buttocks. Brown fat tends to be situated deeper inside the body.

The ability of brown fat to produce heat is called thermogenesis. As you eat more calories, the brown fat balances the intake by converting fat into heat and so burning more fat. If the brown fat is fairly active you will be less likely to store yellow fat. Slim people seem to possess the most effective brown fat heat-producing ability whereas people who gain weight don't seem to be so good at it.

Thermogenesis can be stimulated by thyroid hormone. So when your thyroid is working efficiently, you are usually warm and have warm hands and feet; when it isn't you may feel cold. That is why it is well worth taking your basal body temperature as described earlier in this chapter to see whether your body temperature is too low.

Hysterectomy

Weight gain can often follow a hysterectomy. Women sometimes put on at least 12.7kg (2 stone) after this operation. It could be hormonal, it could be emotional – the cause is uncertain.

Prescribed drugs

Weight gain is often linked to certain medication such as HRT, the contraceptive pill and steroids. Certain anti-depressants can also cause increased appetite and weight gain. If you have to take medication discuss your weight problem with your doctor and ask if there are alternative drugs you could take. On no account should you stop taking medication without guidance from your GP.

FOOD ALLERGIES

The term food allergy has been used to describe an adverse reaction to a particular food. It is thought that all allergies involve an immune system response. For some people this response is almost immediate. Common foods that are linked to this type of allergy are shellfish, some seeds, strawberries and, more severely, peanuts. Symptoms can range from a rash to, more unpleasantly, a slight fever, diarrhoea or constipation. In extreme cases, the allergy can cause a serious reaction which can close up the airways and this requires urgent medical attention. This is known as anaphylactic shock and, fortunately, is not common.

The less acute reactions are known as masked food allergies or slow acting allergies. They don't cause illness and seldom are they bad enough to warrant a GP visit, yet they can generate regular minor symptoms which are often attributed to all sorts of things other than food. These symptoms include bloating of the abdomen, water retention (on fingers, knees and face), digestive disorders, aching joints, fatigue, stuffy nose, skin problems, hyperactivity, headaches and weight gain.

So how can you tell if you have a food allergy?

A good clue would be if you crave a particular food that you eat frequently. Have you noticed when you've been on holiday abroad that you really miss, to the point of being agitated, a certain food that you enjoy at home? If the answer is 'yes' then also ask yourself if it is the same food you have most trouble giving up whenever you try to lose weight? If the answer is 'yes' again then perhaps your body is trying to tell you something. Once a food allergy exists the food becomes mildly addictive and you can be compelled to eat beyond your energy requirements. It's worth considering whether it's this which is hindering your weight loss. Also, if your body's immune system is 'fighting' the foods it is allergic to it is likely to be operating less effectively in other areas.

How can you track down a food allergy?

You can do two possible things. Either have a blood test done (this is explained fully in Chapter 8) or put yourself on the hypo-allergenic diet (described below) for two weeks during which you stop eating all the foods and drinks which are known to be linked to food allergies.

THE HYPO-ALLERGIC DIET

The diet is reproduced here by kind permission of the Society for the Promotion of Nutritional Therapy.

You May Eat
All fresh vegetables
Includes raw, frozen but not tinned, lightly steamed or stewed vegetables, salads, soups made with fresh vegetables, potatoes (without butter).

All fresh fruits and pure fruit juices
Tinned fruit is allowed occasionally so long as it is in natural juice with no added sugar.

All fresh or frozen fish
Oily fish like mackerel, herrings and sardines are especially recommended. Tinned fish is acceptable if in pure oil, brine or spring water.

All unsalted fresh or roasted nuts and seeds
Includes almonds, Brazils, walnuts, cashews, hazelnuts and pecans. Sesame seeds and linseeds need to be ground up first otherwise they just pass straight through you. Other seeds to include are sunflower seeds, pumpkin seeds, pine kernels. Tahini (sesame seed paste) and other nut butters are fine as long as they are sugar and additive free.

All pulses
Includes lentils, chickpeas, kidney beans, butter beans, peanuts, haricot beans, aduki beans. You can cook these yourself or buy canned so long as they do

not contain sugar or anything else except salted water. If you are cooking kidney beans and chick peas remember they need to be soaked overnight. The water should then be discarded and the beans cooked thoroughly in fresh water.

All soya products
Includes tofu and soya milk but not soy sauce as it contains wheat and sometimes contains MSG (monosodium glutamate). Use wheat-free tamari instead.

All cold pressed (unrefined) oils
Includes sesame, sunflower, extra virgin olive oil. The supermarket oils (except extra virgin olive oil) often contain added chemicals and should be avoided.

Non-gluten grains
Includes brown rice, millet and buckwheat as well as flours and flakes made from these grains. Since grains are very small, they can absorb more pesticide, so try to buy them organically grown if available. Use arrowroot or cornflour as thickeners.

Natural sweeteners
Includes honey (in small amounts), maple syrup, rice syrup, date syrup. Pure herbal or fruit teas.

You may not eat (*You will need to read all food labels carefully*)

Dairy products
All cow, sheep and goat products including butter, cheese, milk, yoghurt or anything containing dairy products, lactose or whey.

Gluten grains
Wheat, oats and any others except those on the 'allowed' list above. Look out for these grains in bread, pastry, sauces, gravies, pasta, batter, cakes or biscuits.

Stock cubes and powders, gravy and sauce mixes
These can contain disguised wheat (in the form of hydrolysed vegetable protein) or yeast. Use miso paste dissolved in hot water and add to the dish but do not boil once the miso is added because it kills the beneficial effect.

Animal products
Red meat, poultry, eggs.

Stimulants
Sugar, tea, coffee, alcohol, sweets or chocolate.

Artificial additives
Includes all colourings and preservatives which means you also eliminate 'instant' or convenience foods.

Yeast
Yeast extracts like Marmite, fermented foods like vinegar, sauces and drinks (except miso or tamari). Do check labels.

In the hypo-allergenic diet there is no restriction on the quantity of food you eat, only on the types, and you must stick to the regime or you will undermine the whole purpose. Be organised so that you are well stocked with the foods you are allowed. Try to follow this diet at a time when you have some degree of control over your meals and not too many social events pending. Eat when you need to and don't feel deprived. Keep it up for two weeks if you possibly can, although you may still get good results if you can only follow it for a week.

You must persevere during the first few days when you may feel slightly unwell as your body experiences withdrawal symptoms from certain stimulants such as tea and coffee. You may even develop flu-like symptoms such as headaches, general aches and pains and even diarrhoea. But the result is worth the discomfort – most people say their energy has increased after completing this diet. That's not surprising as their body is no longer diverting energy to battle with foods that didn't agree with it.

What happens when you have finished the hypo-allergenic diet?

If you have completed the hypo-allergenic diet you can now find out what is causing your weight gain and food allergy symptoms. This is done by what is known as food challenging – you begin by returning one type of food from the 'You may not eat' list (e.g. wheat) to your diet for one day only. Then stop eating wheat and monitor yourself for two or three days. Note how you are feeling. Do you feel bloated or tired? Do you have joint pains? Is there any difference?

If you notice a return to your old symptoms after reintroducing wheat then stop eating it as this could indicate that wheat is your problem. However, if at the end of the three days you still feel well and energised then wheat isn't the food causing you a problem. You should then return another type of food to your diet (e.g. a dairy product) for one day only and monitor yourself for the next two or three days as you did before.

It is a good idea to keep a note of your reaction to each food type. Food challenging is a very effective way to track your food allergies. Continue with foods from the 'You may not eat' list until you have challenged them all.

Your pulse rate and food allergies

If you are not sure of your reaction to a particular food you can double check by taking your pulse. It has been found that food allergy or intolerance can cause an increase in pulse rate – as much as ten beats or more.

Pulse test
1. Take your pulse after you have been sitting at rest for a few minutes. The pulse is found on the thumb side of your wrist and you should count how many beats you have in 30 seconds then double your answer to find your pulse rate for one minute.
2. Eat the food that you are challenging and then take your pulse in the same manner ten minutes later. It is valuable to take the pulse again after 30 minutes and then again after one hour. If you have difficulty finding your pulse and counting the beats you could use a heart monitor.

What happens after a blood test for food allergies?

If you've had a blood test then, as with the hypo-allergenic diet, you should have a clear idea of what you are reacting to and can consider whether or not to re-introduce certain foods. If wheat was a problem and you realise it was making you retain weight, then you may decide to eliminate it until you are down to a comfortable size. You could then gradually add wheat, perhaps one slice of toast a day or a portion of pasta, and see whether you feel any different. Most of the time we eat too much of the foods that we are allergic to and overload the body. You may be able to 'get away' with eating some foods if you eat them in moderation.

What happens if you can't link your weight problem to a food allergy?

Don't despair if your failure to lose weight doesn't seem to be linked with any of the reasons given in this chapter. It is actually very good news because it is likely that you will respond well to the natural eating plan outlined in this book. On the positive side, at least you know that you have no undetected food allergies.

CANDIDA

Do you get any of these symptoms?
sugar cravings
cravings for foods such as wine, bread, cheese
migraines or headaches
chronic thrush
inability to lose weight
you feel tired all the time
you wake up feeling tired even after eight hours' sleep
you often feel spaced out
you feel drunk on a small amount of alcohol
you have a bloated, even swollen stomach and excess flatulence?

If you do then you may have a *Candida albicans* overgrowth. We all have the yeast candida in our gut but it is usually controlled by other bacteria. When the immune system is compromised, say because of illness or bad diet, the proportion of the different bacteria can alter, allowing candida to grow out of control.

This overgrowth can also be caused by overuse of antibiotics, use of the contraceptive pill, HRT, steroids and stress – all of which can weaken the immune system.

There is a simple, at-home test for candida overgrowth (see Chapter 8). If you do find you have a candida problem you will need to go on a yeast-free diet and take a course of yeast-free food supplements specifically aimed at eliminating candida. You would be best advised to seek the help of a nutritional therapist.

CHAPTER 6

Get moving – exercise matters

It's a modern day puzzle – we eat fewer calories than we did a hundred years ago and yet we are getting fatter rather than thinner. Why? Well, it can be attributed to many factors such as changes in the type of food we eat, but the main reason for it is the fact that we are now more sedentary.

For our parents' generation exercise was part of the everyday routine and they thought nothing of walking a few miles to and from work. Every household chore required a good deal of effort and was physically demanding: for example, the weekly wash which was done by hand and involved a lot of scrubbing and wringing. In stark contrast, we drive the car to and from the shops, we put the family's clothes in the washing machine and, as for housework, we have endless gadgets to make life easier. Most of us would agree that life is less physically demanding now than it has been for previous generations – the negative result of this is that few of us actually get the exercise our bodies truly need.

Exercise seems to have become a luxury – something to pamper yourself with. Just as you might treat yourself to a new hairstyle or a manicure you might indulge yourself in membership of a smart gym.

We all of us need to make exercise a conscious part of our lives and it doesn't have to cost money. We don't have to join the expensive fitness centre or go to classes.

Instead you could:

- deliberately choose to walk up stairs instead of taking the lift
- walk up escalators
- run, rather than walk, up the stairs at home
- deliberately park the car further away from the shops

None of us would want to go back to the days when the household jobs were an endless, demoralising grind of exhausting physical effort, but we all have to find some way of making up for the lack of everyday exercise in our lives.

Exercise is good for you

The benefits of regular exercise cannot be exaggerated. The older we get, the more important exercise is for our health. Regular exercise has been linked to a lower risk of breast cancer and a higher tolerance of stress. It is absolutely vital for anyone who wants to keep a youthful figure, a good skin and a general zest for life.

Exercise can have a powerful all-round effect on our health. Apart from the feelings of well-being, there are other physical benefits. Moderate exercise performed at a time of day other than just before bed helps improve sleep quality and can also help with insomnia. Exercise helps to keep your bowels working efficiently, which means you are eliminating waste products your body doesn't need. It also improves the function of the immune system, the lymph system and the ability of the body to keep blood sugar in balance. It stimulates thyroid gland secretion and helps to improve thyroid function which has a direct effect on the metabolism. This is especially important if you have an underactive thyroid (see Chapter 5).

Metabolism

We are all governed by our metabolic rate which is exclusive to us. That's why some eating plans might work for a friend but not for you. Understanding and getting to know your metabolism can help you with weight loss and maintenance.

An athletic person who has a high ratio of muscle to fat will have a higher metabolic rate than a person of the same weight with a lower muscle-to-fat ratio. This is because it takes more calories to maintain muscle tissue than fat tissue so the high-ratio athlete will be able to eat more calories than the low-ratio person without gaining weight.

Some people are fortunate enough to be born with a metabolism that causes them little trouble but others aren't. There are times in most slimmers' lives when their metabolism becomes the enemy within. But exercise can help because it boosts the metabolism and allows you to burn fat more efficiently. This means that you are burning off calories at a faster rate than if you did no exercise at all. Studies have shown that the metabolic rate remains higher for at least fifteen hours after exercising.[1]

What is the best exercise for weight loss?

Research shows that long duration, low impact exercise, such as walking or swimming, has a greater benefit on weight loss than short duration, high impact exercise, such as jogging or aerobics. A greater proportion of fat is used when the exercise intensity is low and when we are getting a good supply of oxygen. This means that even while we are exercising we must continue to breathe easily and not puff and pant.

It's the lack of oxygen that causes an excess of lactic acid in the muscles and gives a burning sensation during high impact exercise. Lactic acid inhibits the mobilisation of fat as an energy source – therefore if not enough oxygen is available or the intensity of exercise is too high, fat will not be used. The Health Education Authority is now recommending 30 minutes of moderate exercise, like walking, five times a week. Previously they had recommended 20 minutes of high intensity exercise three times a week.

Walking is one of the best exercises we can choose and probably the simplest to organise. It is also free! To make the walking a bit more taxing, you can put small weights on to your ankles which are attached by Velcro.

How many calories do everyday activities burn in 20 minutes?

Activity	Calories burned
Ironing	20
Housework	60
Mowing the lawn	60
Digging the garden	100
Walking	160
Running upstairs	200

• How does this compare to 20 minutes of various sports?

Sport	Calories burned
Running	240
Cycling	240

Tennis	160
Golf	100
Swimming	240

Emotions

Exercise releases brain chemicals called endorphins which help us to feel happier, more alert and calmer. These have a dramatically positive effect on people suffering from depression, stress, anxiety and insomnia and exercise is often recommended as part of the treatment for these problems.

A study in the *British Medical Journal* in 1985 showed that when half of a group in hospital for depression were asked to do one hour of aerobic exercise three times a week for nine weeks, their depression scores were significantly lower than the other half of the group who did no exercise.[2]

Therefore if you know that you are prone to over-eating when you are stressed, anxious or depressed use exercise to change your mood and lift yourself out of this vicious cycle.

Appetite

As well as releasing feel-good endorphins exercise stimulates other brain chemicals. Corticotropin releasing factor (CRF), for instance, suppresses appetite so that after exercise you simply don't want to stuff yourself with food even though you have burned off plenty of calories. Even when this effect wears off you will find that your body doesn't want unhealthy food. This is because another brain chemical, a neurotransmitter called neuropeptide, which is also released by regular exercise, increases your need for carbohydrates. It 'tells' your body what kind of fuel it needs. When exercise depletes the body's store of energy it will select carbohydrates because they are the primary source of new energy.

You will find that you will quite naturally develop a desire for such things as rice, potatoes, wheat, rye and oats. Just make sure you don't cover them in fats or sugar!

So when you exercise, which uses up energy, your body releases brain chemicals to make you eat more of the foods that replace that energy. It's a very clever system that demonstrates yet again how your body, given the chance, will find the right balance and get you to your correct weight.

Your love life

When you are full of energy and vitality you will be much more interested in sex. Perhaps sometimes you feel you are just too tired for it but by doing exercise you will find that your sex life will be re-energised – all you've got to do is make that initial effort and find the energy to exercise. Once the right chemicals start flowing, so will the romance!

Holidays are a good example. You relax from the normal pressures, you swim, go walking, maybe go dancing and suddenly you find you have energy for things you would be far too tired for at home – including sex. Why wait for a holiday for this to happen? Get yourself fit and active so that you'll enjoy making love regularly. The exercise and good eating will help you to lose weight and you will be more confident about your body, which will also help your love life.

Sex itself could be classed as a form of exercise, as it increases the heart rate and it has been estimated to have the equivalent benefit of a good run around the block.

Heart

Exercise increases the circulation and also seems to lower LDL which is low density lipoprotein (the 'bad' cholesterol) and increase HDL, high density lipoprotein (the 'good' cholesterol). This means the blood can circulate freely instead of becoming obstructed. Regular exercise can help to reduce blood pressure, one of the main risk factors for heart disease, and is especially good for varicose veins.

Breasts

A fascinating study reported in the September 1994 edition of the *US Journal of the National Cancer Institute*[3] showed that women who exercised for around four hours a week had a 58% lower risk of breast cancer and those who routinely exercised for between one and three hours a week had a 30% lower risk. This investigation compared two groups of women under the age of forty and concluded that their activity patterns were a significant predictor of breast cancer risk. What the researchers did not know was pre-cisely why.

It is thought that regular exercise modifies a woman's hormonal activity in a beneficial way. We know that extremes of exercise alter the menstrual cycle dramatically – many athletes and ballet dancers, for instance, don't have periods at all. The suggestion therefore is that moderate, routine exercise suppresses the production, or over-production, of the female hormones, which reduces a woman's exposure to them during her lifetime. As the researchers pointed out, exercise is a good way for women to protect themselves from adolescence onwards. Their research supports the belief that oestrogen may be implicated in breast cancer.

Stress

Do you eat inappropriately when you are stressed? The chances are that you do because you are only human and it's a very natural reaction. One way of controlling this situation is to use exercise as an outlet for your stress.

Exercise helps to keep the adrenal glands healthy. Perched on top of the kidneys, the adrenals secrete the stress hormones adrenaline and noradrenaline (norepinephrine) – both of which should only be brought into play when you are in a 'fight or flight' situation. At a time of danger these chemicals click in and various functions of the body are alerted and modified to prepare you for the impending threat. All this happens very quickly and should only last long enough to get you out of danger.

Our modern lifestyles create stress in the shape of traffic jams, late trains, missed appointments, rudeness, crowds, money worries, work and family upsets. These all take their toll and your body stress responses will come into play. In a 'fight or flight' situation you are naturally prepared to take physical action but in, for example, a traffic jam, you just sit and seethe.

Nowadays people often live in a state of stress which means constant demands are made on the adrenal glands to the point where they can become exhausted. Every day there are numerous instances where the body is put on biochemical 'red alert'.

Stress makes you want to eat (and usually the wrong things), but the stress itself causes the digestive system to be less efficient, so you end up storing that excess food instead of burning it off as energy. If the body has no physical outlet for all this inactive stress, you can suffer symptoms like backache, shoulder pain, tension headaches, digestive problems, ulcers and high blood pressure.

Bones

Astronauts lose bone density in the weightlessness of space because there is no pressure on their bones. The same principle applies to the rest of us – if we don't make demands on our bones they will weaken. This is true for both sexes but particularly for women as they pass the menopause and face the risk of osteoporosis. In fact the bone mass of both men and women decreases naturally as they get older. Women reach their peak bone mass by the time they are 35 so it is important to build as much of it before then as possible. The rate of decline in bone mass increases around the time of the menopause but then slows again.

Use it, don't lose it

If we make demands on our body to provide us with good strong bones then our bone density will be maintained or increased. We can do this by making sure our lives contain a fair amount of physical exercise, either through our lifestyle or through organised exercise.

When the bones are put under stress by use and their strength is in demand, the body draws bone builders called osteoblasts to those areas to build them up. If we become inactive and make no demands on our bones, we are compromising our bone health.

Exercises to put stress on bones include:

- weight-lifting
- brisk walking
- running
- tennis
- badminton
- stair climbing
- aerobics

Not forgetting the everyday activities:

- housework
- shopping
- gardening
- decorating

Every physical activity is better than none. Couch potatoes don't just gain weight, they also allow their bone density to drain away. We all become more frail as we age and some loss of bone density is inevitable. However, through exercise you can keep this loss to a minimum. Women should be especially careful about bone density because their risk of fractures can increase later on in life.

Several studies have shown that weight-bearing exercise helps women maintain or even increase their bone density through and beyond the menopause.[4]

The impact of exercise on bone has been dramatically illustrated by research that examined the difference between the two arms of professional tennis players. The bones of the racket-holding arm, which does most of the work, can be over one third denser than those of the other arm.[5]

General well-being

Exercise keeps our reflexes sharp and improves co-ordination, and the importance of these increase as you pass the 40 landmark. As we get older our range of movement automatically becomes limited unless we make the effort through exercise to maintain it. Stumbles, falls, misjudging steps, turning too quickly can all lead to injuries which may never have happened if we had kept ourselves exercised. Exercise also helps build up muscles, which at any age is important because they act as the first line of defence in shielding our bones from damage.

Can you have too much exercise?

The answer is yes. Too much exercise can cause a change in the body-fat ratio and in women can stop periods. Very young female gymnasts and athletes have found that over-exercising has prevented their periods from even beginning. Most of us, of course, come nowhere near to over-exercising but some people become addicted to exercise, very often those who have had eating problems when they were younger.

HOW TO DESIGN YOUR OWN EXERCISE PROGRAMME

As regular exercise is more beneficial than occasional bursts, it is best to find something you enjoy which will motivate you to do it regularly. Brisk walking is very beneficial and can be fitted in at any time. It does not require special equipment or clothing and costs nothing. As well as being a low impact exercise and therefore excellent for weight loss, it also frees the mind so that your imagination can just 'wander off' while you walk. This can help to alleviate emotional or stress problems. If you have not exercised for a while, walking is a very good way to start getting fit.

Don't rush on to the tennis court if you haven't played for years, or suddenly begin any aerobic type of exercise if you know you are even a little unfit. It's a sure recipe for a nasty muscle injury or even worse. If you have not been exercising regularly, take things slowly at first and build up gradually.

Your pulse rate

Your pulse rate is a good indicator of how fit you are and can help you to know if you are overdoing it when exercising. The more unfit you are, the faster your pulse is, because the heart has to work harder to pump blood around your body.

Find the pulse in your wrist by placing three fingertips on the bone running down from your thumb. Move your fingers inwards until you feel the beat of your pulse. Count the number of beats over thirty seconds and then double your answer to get your pulse per minute.

The maximum your pulse rate should be is 220 minus your age. So if you are 45, your maximum pulse rate is 220 − 45 = 175.

When you are exercising for weight loss, it is suggested that you keep your pulse rate at 65% of this maximum. Check your pulse after three to four minutes of exercise. If your goal was to improve your fitness then your heart rate should be higher than this, but when you want to burn off fat, a steady heart rate of 65% of your maximum is the most efficient way to do so. There are simple heart rate monitors on the market which are worn on the wrist like a watch so it is easy to keep within the correct range for fat loss. 'Staying in Touch' on page 192 of this book gives information on where to buy a heart rate monitor.

Regardless of how fit you feel, if you have a heart or respiratory problem or you are over 50, it is wise to have a general GP check-up before beginning an exercise regime.

Choose an exercise that fits in with your lifestyle

How we exercise is very much a matter of personal choice. We are all individuals so we have to find an exercise routine that fits in with our families, our lifestyle and our finances. Some people prefer to exercise on their own, while others need the motivation of a group or a friend to keep them going. Use whichever way suits you best so that you are more likely to keep active and fit in the long term. Don't be a five-minute wonder!

Body shape

One of the best ways of re-shaping the body is to use resistance training. Research has found that the less muscle you have, the harder it is to lose weight, because muscle is metabolically active but body fat is inactive. Therefore when women diet, but don't exercise, 25% of any weight lost is made up of water, muscle, bone and other lean tissue. Muscle mass uses up more calories than fat: up to 30 to 50 calories a day compared with only 2 calories a day for fat.

Exercise physiologists have found that the best fat-loss exercise programme is a combination of both cardiovascular and resistance training. Some studies have shown that over an 8-week period 30 minutes of exercise a day, split half and half between cardiovascular and resistance training, compared with 30 minutes of purely cardiovascular gave an extra 3kg (7lbs) of fat loss. Research also shows that resistance traing increases metabolism.

In order to get the best results, choose a cardiovascular activity that you enjoy, such as walking, and remember that fat can only be burned in the presence of oxygen. So no going for the burn! Low intensity, long duration is better for fat loss than short, high intensity activities.

Resistance training includes lifting weights, callisthenics or using resistance machines in the gym. There are simple ways of doing this without the need for expensive equipment or even having to join a gym. You only need to invest in a set of dumbbells which are available in varying weights: some people have used rice- or sand-filled bags to get a similar effect. Start with the lowest weight dumbbell and increase over time as you become stronger. You do not need to lift enormous weights, the idea is simply to create a resistance against which your muscles have to work, thereby increasing muscle mass.

For recommended exercises see pages 122-5.

A TYPICAL RESISTANCE PROGRAMME

This set of 6 exercises (continued over the page) will help you to burn off fat because weight training increases the metabolism. Use a set of dumbells for each exercise (or you could use rice-, or sand-filled bags, or even a couple of food cans). Do a number of repetitions (e.g. 10) for each exercise, and then rest for two or three minutes before repeating the set two more times.

Take great care to do the exercises properly rather than fighting with weights that are too heavy. When using weights for the first time, always use the lightest weight available.

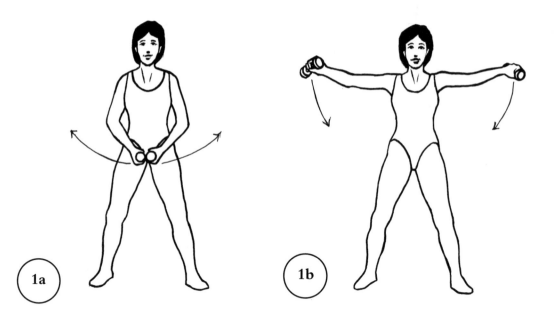

Exercise 1: **Lateral Rise**

The arms should be raised only to shoulder level and the elbows kept bent to take the load of the elbow joint.

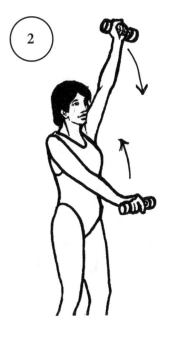

Exercise 2: **Alternate Arm Raise**
Raise each arm alternately in front of the body while keeping the elbows and knees slightly bent. Take care not to arch your back.

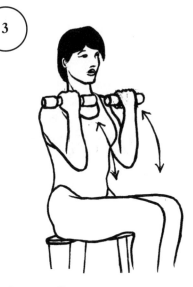

Exercise 3: **Curls**
These can be done in either the seated or standing position and with arms together or alternately.

With strength training, although the exercises seems light the accumulative effect means that you will not only lose weight, especially fat, but also have a more shapely body.

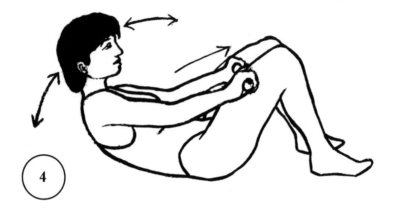

Exercise 4: **Abdominal Crunch**

Lie on your back with your knees raised. While doing the crunches keep the lower back supported on the floor, don't arch the back. Aim the dumbells towards the knees during the lift.

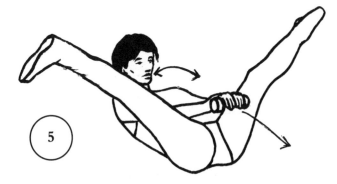

Exercise 5: **Abdominal Crunch Through the Legs**
Lie on your back with your legs raised in the air and wide apart. Pass the dumbells through the open legs.

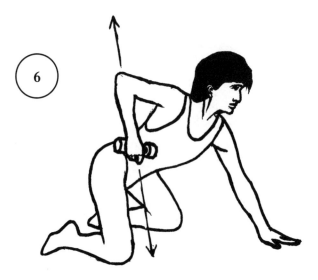

Exercise 6: **One Arm Bent**
On your knees, supporting the body by resting on one arm on the floor, slightly in front of your shoulders. Pull the weight to the shoulder without arching the back.

Being fit is more important than being thin

Being clinically obese is a health risk but recent research is showing that a person's level of fitness is the most important factor in terms of health.

Professor Stephen Blair of the Dallas Laboratories in America has been studying 25,000 people of varying ages, shapes and sizes since 1970 . Over eight years he has found that more people die who are unfit but of normal weight than people who are fit but overweight.

Make health your goal

You will find, as many others have done, that on the road to becoming fit and enjoying the pleasure of food, you will automatically lose fat. If you make health your goal rather than the losing of weight, your whole perspective on food will change and you'll find you achieve your appropriate weight without being on endless diets.

CHAPTER 7

Still need more help with weight loss?

Even though you will lose weight if you follow the guidelines in this book you are bound to wonder if there is anything further you can do to nudge the scales in the right direction. You might consider complementary medicine. All slimmers need as much help as they can get during the gradual journey to their ideal weight. Complementary medicine can be extremely useful in helping to improve metabolism, maintaining a stable appetite, eliminating cravings, detoxifying your body and generally getting you into optimum health by restoring balance throughout the body.

NUTRITIONAL THERAPY

Food is, and should be, regarded as a powerful medicine – it has a huge impact on the biochemical processes of the body. Nutritional therapy is not just about eating well but also about correcting any vitamin or mineral deficiencies. You need to eat a good variety of food so as to give yourself the best chance of getting all the nutrients you need.

How can supplements help?

Vitamins and minerals work in harmony and most of them are dependent on each other in order to act efficiently. The best way to structure a supplement programme for yourself is to take a good combined multi-vitamin and mineral supplement. You can then add in other supplements if you feel you need to.

A number of chemical reactions are involved to turn glucose into energy instead of fat. These are controlled by enzymes, which are themselves dependent on certain vitamins and minerals in the body. If these are deficient, you will lack energy and feel low and that will make it more difficult for your body to turn glucose into energy instead of storing it as fat. You can help yourself by taking a good balance of vitamins and minerals in supplement form. There are also some nutrients which are extremely helpful in getting rid of that extra weight while you are sorting out your new eating plan and exercise programme. Remember, these aids aren't instead of eating appropriately, they are in addition to it!

If you have been yo-yo dieting for a number of years, either restricting food intake or trying different diet drinks or pills, it is likely that you are deficient in a number of vitamins and minerals. Supplements could certainly help if you know you've been depriving yourself for a long time, possibly even years. Nowadays a lot of our food is refined and therefore stripped of valuable nutrients – even the soil our food grows in is depleted of vitamins and minerals through overuse.

There are twenty-two vitamins and minerals which are essential for the control of our weight and metabolism. The most important ones are vitamins B2, B3, B5, B6 and C, choline, inositol, chromium, manganese and zinc.

When it comes to buying food supplements you get what you pay for. I would recommend buying capsules rather than tablets. Capsules tend to be filled only with active ingredients while tablets can include a variety of fillers, binders and bulking agents. So it's important to read the labels. Excellent supplement companies are BioCare, Lamberts and Nutrizec.

VITAMINS

Vitamins are essential for life and are required in very small amounts for healthy growth and development. The body is unable to make them for itself so it is vital that you include them either within the food you eat or in supplement form. Supplements are *not* a substitute for food and have no calorie or energy value of their own.

The B vitamins are important; they are often called the 'stress' vitamins because of their ability to help us cope with pressures in everyday life. Vitamins B3 and B6 are especially important as they help to supply fuel to cells ready for burning for energy. Vitamin B6 is necessary, together with zinc, for the production of pancreatic enzymes which help our effective digestion of food. If our digestion is good then we will efficiently use up our food instead of storing it as fat.

Vitamins B2, B3 and B6 are necessary for normal thyroid hormone production, so any deficiencies in these can affect thyroid function and consequently affect the metabolism. B3 is also a component of the glucose tolerance factor (GTF) which is released every time blood sugar rises.

Vitamin B5 has also been shown to help with weight loss. In one test a hundred people, aged between 15 and 55, were given 2.5g of B5 in pantothenic acid form, four times a day and they all reported an average weight loss of 1.2kg (2.75lbs) per week. The researchers suggested that a deficiency of vitamin B5 reduces our ability to utilise fat.[1] Vitamin B5 (pantothenic acid) plays an important role in energy production and is also necessary for optimum adrenal function.

To ensure you get a good supply of B vitamins the easiest way is to take a B complex along with a good multi-vitamin and mineral supplement.

Vitamin C can play a role in weight control too. It helps to lower cholesterol and is involved in the conversion of glucose to energy in the cells.

Vitamins that help weight loss and where to find them

Vitamin – B2 (riboflavin)
Function
Turns fat, sugar and protein into energy. Needed for hair, nails and eyes.
Good sources
Almonds, wild rice, soya beans, broccoli, wholemeal bread, mackerel, eggs, yoghurt

Vitamin – B3 (niacin)
Function
Needed for energy production. Balances blood sugar. Controls cholesterol balance.
Good sources
Canned tuna in oil, salmon, wholewheat, asparagus, almonds, brown rice

Vitamin – B5 (pantothenic acid)
Function
Involved in energy production, controls fat metabolism
Good sources
Wholewheat, alfalfa sprouts, peas, lentils, eggs, mushrooms, brown rice

Vitamin – B6 (pyridoxine)
Function
Helps with digestion of protein. Important in maintaining hormone balance. Useful for PMS and as an anti-depressant.
Good sources
Brown rice, cauliflower, grilled herring, soya beans, sweet potatoes, sunflower seeds

Vitamin – C (ascorbic acid)
Function
Needed to make collagen for healthy bones, skin, muscles and joints. Critical to immune function and an important antioxidant. Turns food into energy.
Good sources
Raw peppers, broccoli, cauliflower, strawberries, peas, baked potatoes, oranges

Vitamin – Choline
Function
Member of the B complex family and required for the correct metabolism of fats. Without it fats can block metabolism by becoming trapped in the liver.
Good sources
Eggs, cauliflower, cucumber, peanuts

Vitamin – Inositol
Function
Works closely with choline and again helps to transport fat from the liver.
Good sources
Soya, eggs, citrus fruits, wholegrains, nuts

MINERALS

Minerals are contained in the soil and are absorbed by plants and, in turn, anything that eats those plants which includes us and the animals we eat. Unfortunately over time the soil has been depleted of some of these minerals and so there are now much fewer in the plants we eat than a generation ago.

Mineral supplements like calcium should be in the form of citrates, ascorbates or polynicotinates which are more easily absorbed by the body. Chlorides, sulphates, carbonates and oxides should be avoided since they are not so easily assimilated and therefore mineral supplements in this form may pass through the body without being absorbed. The other way minerals are made more digestible is by chelation (pronounced 'keylation'). Chelated minerals allow three to ten times greater assimilation than the non-chelated ones, so watch out for that word on labels.

Zinc

Zinc is an important mineral in appetite control and a deficiency can cause a loss of taste and smell, creating a need for stronger tasting foods including more salty, sugary and/or spicy foods. Zinc also functions together with vitamins A and E in the manufacture of thyroid hormone.

Chromium

Chromium has been the most widely researched mineral with regard to its effectiveness as an aid to weight loss. Chromium is needed for the metabolism of sugar and without it insulin is less effective in controlling blood sugar levels. It is the major nutrient in glucose tolerance factor (GTF). It also helps to control levels of fat and cholesterol in the blood. One study showed that people who took chromium picolinate over a ten week period lost an average of 1.9kg (4.2lb) of fat while those on a placebo lost only 0.2kg (0.4lb).[2]

If you are diabetic then you need to speak to your doctor before supplementing with chromium.

Manganese

This mineral helps with the metabolism of fats and helps to stabilise blood sugar. It also functions in many enzyme systems including enzymes involved in energy metabolism and thyroid hormone function.

Minerals that help weight loss and where to find them

Zinc
Function
Necessary for correct action of many hormones including insulin, so important in balancing blood sugar. Also necessary for fertility.
Good sources
Oysters, pumpkin seeds, wholewheat, rye, oats, almonds, peas

Chromium
Function
Active component of glucose tolerance factor (GTF). Maintains blood sugar balance. Controls cravings and reduces hunger.
Good sources
Wholewheat bread, rye bread, potatoes, apples, eggs, parsnips, carrots

Manganese

Function

Balances blood sugar and is important for metabolism and healthy thyroid function which is essential in maintaining a healthy weight.

Good sources

Almonds, rye, wholewheat, oats, Brussels sprouts, carrots

OTHER USEFUL SUPPLEMENTS

Co-enzyme Q10

This supplement is important for energy production. It's found in all the tissues and organs of our bodies. As we get older we may become deficient which results in a reduction of energy and a slowing down of the life-giving process. It has been used to help heart problems, high blood pressure, gum disease and immune deficiencies.[3]

A study also showed that people on a low-fat diet doubled their weight loss when supplemented with Q10 compared to those who did not take it.[4] While a low-fat diet is not advocated, it does show that, of two groups of people on the same diet, the ones taking Q10 benefited.

It can be bought in tablet form from a good health food shop.

Garcinia cambogia

A small tropical fruit called the Malabar tamarind can also help with weight loss. It originates in central Asia, where the rind is used in Thai and Indian cooking. The garcinia contains HCA (hydroxy-citric acid), which is related to the citric acid found in citrus fruits and which can enable carbohydrates to be turned into usable energy instead of being deposited as fat. The HCA in this fruit seems to curb appetite, reduce food intake and inhibit the formation of fat and cholesterol. Unlike some appetite suppressants, it achieves this effect without stimulating the central nervous system so is more healthy for us.

Instead of making fats and cholesterol which would normally occur after a meal, HCA encourages the body to make more glucose, which can be burned as energy instead. The brain monitors the levels of glucose and glycogen (glucose stores) in the liver. When they are low the brain signals 'hunger' and we feel the need to eat again. With HCA most of our last meal will have been used to make glucose and so the liver will give the signal that the glucose level is OK, making it longer before we feel the need to eat again.

This plays a key role in both carbohydrate and fat metabolism and results in fats and LDL (bad) cholesterol being reduced.[5]

Other research has shown that HCA may help increase the rate at which we burn fat. The theory is that it activates an enzyme called carnitine acetyltransferase which speeds up the fat-burning process.

In one trial 50 overweight people were given a low-fat diet to follow. Those who also took HCA lost nearly three times the weight of those who didn't.

Garcinia cambogia is usually marketed under the name Citrimax and is available in health food shops and chemists. BioCare, a good supplement company, combines HCA with chromium (marketed as Citrimax Plus) which is an excellent combination. Another supplement called VitaTrim from Nutrizec combines *Garcinia cambogia* with chromium and L-carnitine. The amino acid L-carnitine plays an active part in the fat-burning process and has also been used to lower cholesterol and triglycerides. 'Staying in touch' on page 191 of this book tells you how to get hold of these supplements if you cannot obtain them locally.

Soya

The value of adding soya to your eating plan has been discussed in Chapter 3 and you can include it in the form of soya milk, tofu, soya sauce, miso, etc. Because we have not been brought up eating soya some people find the taste hard to get used to. Soya is a valuable food and if you have difficulty eating it you might consider taking it as a supplement. It can be bought in health food shops containing both of the soya isoflavones – genistein and daidzein.

Tryptophan

As mentioned in Chapter 1 scientists are looking into the possibility of adding tryptophan to everyday foods to help people feel less depressed when they reduce their food intake to lose weight. It is worrying to think that our freedom to choose what we are eating may be challenged by this. Tryptophan is an essential amino acid and it occurs naturally in foods such as dairy products, meat, fish, turkey, bananas, dried dates and peanuts, but of course, when you used to diet and reduced your intake of many of these foods, you also reduced your levels of tryptophan which helps to produce serotonin, a brain chemical that governs mood (see Chapter 2).

Until 1990, l-tryptophan was bought as a food supplement for help with insomnia, anxiety and depression. Then a Japanese biotech company produced a genetically engineered tryptophan which was implicated in 37 deaths. In 1997, a new product arrived in the UK called 5-hydroproxytryptophan (5-HTP) which originated from a small African bean called *Griffonia simplicifolia*. The bean had attracted the attention of scientists because it contained an amino acid, 5-hydroproxytryptophan, which in the body converts naturally to the brain chemical serotonin.

Researchers from the Psychiatry Department at Belgium's University of Stuivenberg have shown that giving clinically depressed patients 5-HTP increased their beta-endorphin (a feel-good brain chemical) concentrations significantly compared with that of patients on a placebo and improved their clinical diagnosis.

NB *It is very important that you check with your doctor before taking any form of tryptophan as it can be potentially dangerous for anyone taking mono-amine oxidase inhibitor (MAOI) drugs for depression.*

HELP WITH CELLULITE

That 'orange peel' effect on the skin is notoriously difficult to eliminate. It is found mostly on the thighs and unfortunately affects women almost to the exclusion of men because of a difference in cell structure between men and women. The tissue that is affected in cellulite is the subcutaneous tissue just below the surface of the skin. When women's thighs are pinched, we get a pitting and bulging effect, but when men's thighs are pinched, their skin folds or furrows instead. Doesn't seem fair, does it?

Although it is often said that cellulite is caused by accumulation of waste products, it is more likely to be a problem with fat cells. It is more common in obesity and during the menopause when connective tissue can become thinner, allowing the fat cells to become bigger. Anything that helps restore connective tissue is going to be helpful. As discussed in Chapter 6 regular exercise can be very helpful in improving the appearance of the cellulite.

You might try:
Gota kola (*Centella asiatica*) is a herb that is helpful in the battle against cellulite and has produced impressive results in clinical trials.[6] It has also been shown to increase the circulation in the legs and to help with varicose veins.

Body brushing encourages lymphatic drainage and removal of toxins from the body. In so doing it helps to reduce, even eliminate, cellulite in areas such as the thighs and buttocks, where protein, fats and waste materials tend to accumulate. Also, as you change your way of eating and your body starts to re-balance itself, you will release the excess toxins and waste products that your body was holding on it. Daily body brushing is a gentle yet powerful way to help encourage the detoxification process.

How to body brush

Using a natural fibre brush and, with your body dry, begin at the tips of your shoulders and cover your whole body, except your head, with long smooth strokes, always brushing towards your heart. At first brush gently as your skin will need to get used to the sensation. It will also go slightly red as you start to increase the circulation in areas which may have become stagnated. Try to do this daily.

Exercise can also help reduce cellulite as it helps restore a slim subcutaneous fat layer. As you lose weight, the cellulite will also reduce but it is important that you do not lose weight rapidly as this can make the appearance of cellulite worse.

Using a special massage oil for cellulite can also be helpful. The Body Shop has one which includes a blend of almond, apricot kernel, mandarin and lemon oils to help smooth the skin. It recommends the cellulite massage oil is used with a loofah or bath mitt and a little salt to tone the problem areas.

HELP FOR A SLUGGISH METABOLISM

If you have any of the symptoms listed in Chapter 5 check with your doctor that you do not have an underactive thyroid. If the thyroid blood tests are fine but your basal body temperatures are low then it is possible that your metabolism is sluggish.

The thyroid gland is like a thermostat which regulates your body temperature by secreting two hormones which control how quickly the body burns calories and uses energy. These hormones are made from iodine and the amino acid tyrosine. Naturally rich sources of iodine are seafoods, especially saltwater fish and seaweeds such as kelp. Tyrosine is found in foods including almonds, avocados, bananas, pumpkin and sesame seeds.

Herbalists have traditionally used bladderwrack, which is a seaweed, to help with an underactive thyroid. This is normally taken as a tablet, but if you are lucky enough to be able to buy it fresh or dried, you can make an infusion by pouring a cup of boiling water on to 10-15ml (2-3 teaspoons) of dried bladderwrack and leaving it for ten minutes. This infusion can be drunk three times a day.

HELP FOR DEPRESSION

If you eat when you are depressed and find it hard to break this vicious circle, then it is worth trying to alleviate the depression naturally.
Try:
St John's wort (*Hypericum*) is a herb that has been widely studied with regard to its success in relieving mild or moderately severe depression with no side effects. A review of 23 clinical trials involving more than 1,750 people published in 1996 in the *British Medical Journal* found the herb to be 'significantly superior' to a placebo and 'similarly effective as standard anti-depressants' including Prozac. St John's wort has been shown to produce improvements in a number of psychological symptoms including depression, anxiety, apathy, sleep disturbances, insomnia and feelings of worthlessness.
Aromatherapy oils can also be very useful in lifting your mood. Both bergamot and neroli oils can be added to a bath or used in a massage oil. Ylang ylang and jasmine also have a powerful euphoric effect. See 'Aromatherapy' on page 144 for various ways to use them.

HELP FOR STRESS

If you eat because you are stressed, then you need to learn to stay calm. Keep detached from the problem to take a step back from the stress. From reading the other sections in this book about stress you will understand the importance of maintaining your blood sugar levels by eating every three hours. There are also natural remedies which can help stress.

For example:
Magnesium is classed as 'nature's tranquilliser' so it is worth adding to your diet in the form of a supplement. The B vitamins (see 'Vitamins' on page 128) are well known for their ability to help with alleviating stress so these too should also be included.

Take daily:
300mg magnesium and vitamin B complex containing 100mg of each B vitamin.

Herbs really come into their own when it comes to trying to control stress and the ones specifically stress-related are called nervines. They act on the nervous system to relieve anxiety, tension and irritability and one of the most well-known is valerian. It is most effective when combined with skullcap which also relaxes the nervous system and at the same time can renew a flagging nervous system. Skullcap has been used for pre-menstrual tension too.

Ginseng is also good for anxiety and tension and Korean or Chinese, known as panax, are often used as a tonic since they help the adrenal glands function. Studies have shown that the use of panax ginseng can help us withstand the effects of many different stressful situations, increase our mental alertness and boost vitality and physical performance. Siberian ginseng also helps in stressful situations and has a more subtle effect than panax. Both ginsengs are adaptogens which means they have a normalising, balancing effect on the body.

Aromatherapy can also help with stress and can be used in a bath or rubbed into the back of your neck. Neroli, rose or sandalwood can help calm and relax. If you are feeling irritable then essential oils like camomile, lavender and geranium are good for calming anger as well as balancing the feelings. See 'Aromatherapy' on page 144 for various ways to use them.

HELP FOR WATER RETENTION

Water retention is a common problem and for women is often worst just before a period. It can be so bad you may have trouble getting rings on fingers and shoes on your feet. It can also add a kilo or so to your weight. Your first instinct may be to limit the amount you drink, but in fact you should do the opposite. It's important to drink more water and reduce your intake of salt, including hidden salt in convenience foods. If you limit your intake of water your body will think there is a shortage and try to retain the water you have, hence the swelling in the first place.

Many women who suffer from water retention turn to diuretics. These will increase the rate at which fluid is lost but will also flush important minerals out of the body – for example, potassium, which is vital in the correct functioning of the heart.

Try these natural diuretics:

Dandelion is a natural diuretic that allows fluid to be released without losing vital nutrients at the same time. It contains more vitamins and minerals than any other herb and is one of the best natural sources of potassium. An interesting experiment with animals who were given this herb showed they lost 30% of their original body weight.[7] The researchers felt this was due to the release of water retention. Dandelion can be taken as a tincture or as a decoction of 10-15ml (2-3 teaspoons) of the root in one cup of water (bring it to the boil and then simmer for 10 minutes). Dandelion leaves can also be eaten raw in salads.

Parsley is not only rich in vitamin C, but is a useful diuretic too. It is best taken in tincture form for the diuretic effect but also can be eaten raw.

Aromatherapy can also help water retention, particularly fennel oil. Add ten drops of fennel to a warm bath and lie in it for 15 to 20 minutes. Then massage your body using 15 drops of fennel (see 'Aromatherapy' on page 144 for how to make up a massage oil as it should not be used neat).

HELP YOUR LIVER

This vital gland (the largest in the body) is part of the digestive system. Among its many tasks are the storage and filtration of blood, the secretion of bile and numerous metabolic functions, including the conversion of sugars into glycogen. It plays a vital part in fat metabolism and in the oxidation of fat to produce energy. It's worrying therefore that in many overweight people the liver can be impaired.[8]

Excess food is converted to fat in the liver and then transported around the body to be stored. The liver also plays a part in thyroid function by converting thyroxin into the more active form triiodothyronine. When this conversion is insufficient a person may develop an underactive thyroid (hypothyroidism) which we have looked at in Chapter 5. The liver is also the waste disposal unit of the body. It detoxifies by combining harmful substances like chemicals, drugs and alcohol with less harmful substances which are then excreted by the kidneys.

Certain natural remedies, including herbs, can be used to optimise the functioning of the liver and aid its ability to break down and metabolise fats:

Dandelion has already been mentioned in relation to water retention (page 137) but it is also an important liver herb. It is a gentle tonic for the liver and helps to increase the secretion of bile which assists the digestive system (including the digestion of fat).

Milk thistle (*Silybum marianum*) is another excellent herb for the liver. A number of studies have shown that it can increase the number of new liver cells to replace old damaged ones.[9] Silymarin is the collective name for the substances found in milk thistle which have this beneficial effect and can be taken as a tincture or in capsule form.

Lipotropic agents are substances that stop excessive fat from collecting in the liver. They detoxify the liver and trigger its production of lecithin which emulsifies cholesterol and fat in the bloodstream into smaller, less harmful substances. These lipotropics include choline, inositol and methionine.

Nature supplies us with these agents in the following foods:
Choline – lentils, split peas, rice, lecithin from soya, eggs and wheat germ
Inositol – rice, lentils and barley
Methionine – an essential amino acid found in most abundance in eggs

SEVEN DAY LIVER SPRING CLEAN

The liver, as our waste disposal unit, will only eliminate environmental toxins and waste products properly when it is working efficiently. We need, therefore, to keep it functioning in peak condition, especially when we are losing weight, so that we clear out any excesses. The liver also helps us eliminate 'old' hormones. This is important for both men and women. An excess of oestrogen for women has been linked to breast cancer and an excess of testosterone for men to prostrate cancer.

Here is a very gentle detox regime:
Days 1 and 2:
Cut out tea, coffee and alcohol to prepare your body for the cleanse.

Days 3 to 7:
First thing in the morning, before you have eaten anything, drink this liver 'flush' to help your body get rid of environmental toxins and waste products and give you a spring clean.

In a liquidiser mix:
250ml (8fl oz) freshly squeezed lemon juice
250ml (8fl oz) spring or mineral water
1 fresh garlic clove
1 tablespoon extra virgin olive oil
1cm (½ in) fresh ginger root

If you can't drink all that lemon juice, use organic apple juice instead with a squeeze of lemon. Blend to a smooth liquid and drink slowly.

Drink some apple juice afterwards, if you have an aftertaste, and 15 minutes later drink a cup of hot peppermint tea. Then eat normally but keep your meals very simple so that your body has the chance to eliminate toxins. Eat plenty of fresh fruit and vegetables, salads, stir-fried vegetables, vegetable soups, brown rice, porridge oats, etc. You may have headaches or flu-like symptoms for the first couple of days, which are indications that you are detoxifying. You must eat well to keep your blood sugar up. You can repeat this programme every couple of months if you feel you benefit from it.

HELP WITH CONSTIPATION

There can, of course, be medical reasons for this problem but very often constipation is caused by unhealthy eating. If you are a sufferer you should first increase the amount of fibre in your eating plan (as outlined in Chapter 3). However, while you are changing your eating patterns, you may need some extra help.

Normal laxatives work by stimulating or increasing the number of bowel movements or by encouraging a softer or bulkier stool. Unfortunately they do not address the cause of the problem, such as lack of fibre. It's also possible to become dependent upon them. The more laxatives are used, the less the body has to do for itself and ultimately the bowel can lose its tone and muscle action and cannot function. The other problem with laxatives is that they cause the food to rush out of the body before the vital nutrients have been absorbed.

Herbal laxatives are generally more gentle. Ingredients include butternut, blue flag and psyllium. Their effects are two-fold – first they create a healthy and frequent bowel movement and second they tone the bowel to encourage its own natural function. Good herbal companies have ready-made capsules of a number of gentle bowel-toning herbs and also capsules (or powder) to use for a bowel cleanse to help detoxify the colon. Herbal essences to be taken with water are also available. Your local good health food shop should be able to advise.

THE VALUE OF FIBRE

The importance of eating fibre was emphasised in Chapter 3. While fibre is important in the prevention of colon problems, such as diverticulitis, it also plays a major role in weight loss. The presence of fibre in your eating plan helps to speed up the passage of food through your digestive system. The longer food stays in your intestines, the more calories are being absorbed.

Fibre helps with appetite control because it gives you the 'bulk', helping you to feel more full without the extra calories.

There are two kinds of fibre that we can eat, soluble and insoluble. It is the soluble fibre that gives the feeling of fullness and it will also bind with some of the cholesterol and fat in the food you eat. This helps keep fat levels under control as the fibre passes out unabsorbed. Most plants provide both types but good sources of soluble fibre include oats, pulses and most fruit and vegetables. Good sources of insoluble fibre are rice, nuts and wheat.

You should ideally obtain fibre from the food you eat but, while you are trying to reach your target weight, soluble fibre can be useful taken in supplement form, either capsule, tablet or powder. Once swallowed with water it swells up in the stomach, makes you feel full and can reduce the appetite. Guar gum and psyllium husks are two forms of soluble fibre which can be taken in supplement form; they should be taken with a glass of water approximately fifteen minutes before eating.

One particular type of fibre called glucomannan which comes from the Japanese konjac plant can be very useful as it absorbs more water than most other kinds. There has been one double-blind placebo-controlled study on konjac fibre which showed that over a 12 week period the people on the fibre lost 2.24kg (4.93lb) compared to 0.65kg (1.45lb) on the placebo. In statistical terms this difference was not significant but the konjac fibre may be a useful supplement along with changes in eating patterns and exercise.[10]

FLOWER ESSENCES

Bach Flower Remedies can be used to address the emotional issues around food. Many health food shops sell them and they are easy to use. Just add a few drops of the essence to a glass of water and drink throughout the day.
Crab Apple can remedy low self-image.
Cherry Plum is helpful for alleviating a sense of being out of control around food.
Self-heal and Rock Water can help those who reward and punish themselves with food and who feel physically or emotionally uncomfortable with food.
Morning Glory and St John's Wort can help stop impulsive eating.

VITAMIN E

This vitamin is not directly related to helping weight loss but has been included because it is so beneficial to good health. A study published in *The Lancet* in 1996 by scientists from Cambridge University and Papworth Hospital showed that taking a daily dose of vitamin E reduced the risk of having a heart attack by an astonishing 75%. An 18 month trial involved 2,000 patients with coronary arteriosclerosis (fatty deposits in the arteries). Half of the patients were given the vitamin E supplement with their regular medication and half took the placebo with their regular medication.[11]

Professor Morris Brown, of Cambridge University, commented on this research in the *Journal of the Institute for Optimum Nutrition*:

> This is even more exciting than aspirin. Most people in our study were already taking aspirin. The average benefit from taking aspirin is in the order of 25-40% reduction. Vitamin E reduces the risk of heart attack by a massive 75%.[12]

With heart disease being the biggest killer for both men and women this is very important research, especially as the risk of heart disease increases with weight gain.

Don't we get enough vitamin E from what we eat?

Dr Malcolm Mitchinson, the co-author of the Cambridge study referred to above, believes that even if we eat a well balanced diet it will not give us enough vitamin E to protect us against heart disease. The American Heart Association has also stated that vitamin E is one of the 'top ten heart and stroke research advances for 1996'.

As well as the benefits for the heart, vitamin E can also boost the immune system. Researchers at Tufts University in Boston, USA, have looked at the effects of vitamin E on the immune systems of older people. Eighty-eight volunteers aged 65 and older were divided into four groups. One group was given 60ius of vitamin E a day, the second group 200ius, the third group 800ius and the fourth a placebo. None of the groups knew what they were taking.

After four months the results were very interesting. As we get older our immune cells function less effectively but the groups taking vitamin E seemed to have cells that functioned as if they belonged to younger people. The best results were obtained with the group taking 200ius per day and this may be the optimum dose for the immune system.

Because of this effect on the immune system and the research that is suggesting that free radicals may play a role in the cancer process, vitamin E has been looked at as an anti-oxidant. A number of studies have shown a relationship between low blood levels of vitamin E and the occurrence of certain cancers including breast cancer in women,[13] colon cancer,[14] lung cancer,[15] cervical cancer[15] and mouth cancers.[16]

This amazing vitamin has also been shown to help decrease the risk of developing cataracts,[17] alleviating menopausal hot flushes,[18] slowing down the ageing process[19] and lessening premenstrual symptoms such as bloating and depression.[20]

Good food sources of vitamin E are unrefined oils including corn and sunflower oil, peanuts, sesame seeds and oily fish like tuna, sardines and salmon.

OTHER WAYS OF CONTROLLING APPETITE

Alan Hirsch, of the Smell and Taste Treatment and Research Foundation in Chicago, says that cravings for certain foods are more often about craving aromas. Interestingly 95% of taste comes from smell and only 5% from senses in the mouth. When a smell is sniffed into the nasal cavity it gets dissolved in mucus in special olfactory receptors. An electrical signal is then triggered which travels along nerve fibres into the brain. We are able to smell around 10,000 different chemicals through 500 to 1,000 receptors.

Try a simple experiment:

Close your eyes and pinch your nose, then ask someone to put different foods into your mouth one at a time. See if you can identify what you are eating. You will find this very interesting because it is extremely difficult to tell what you are eating without being able to smell it.

Hirsch found that sniffing fragrances like banana and peppermint helped dieters drop 2.27kg (5lb) or 2% of their total body weight in a month because it seemed to subdue the urge to snack.

Tips from Hirsch include:

- Savour the smell of your food before you eat it
- Eat your food hot
- Chew every mouthful thoroughly

COMPLEMENTARY THERAPIES THAT CAN HELP WITH WEIGHT LOSS PROBLEMS

Herbal medicine

Herbs are the oldest form of medicine and have been used for healing in all cultures and in all times. There are a number of ways they can help with weight loss.

Herbs are in fact the foundation of numerous pharmaceutical drugs; aspirin is based on an extract from willow, originally used for pain relief by the native Americans and steroids have been derived from wild yam. Up to 70% of drugs in use today have their origins in plants, yet modern pharmaceutical practice bears no relation to the ancient tradition of using plants for medicinal purposes. Drug companies use only the active ingredient of the plant or herb in a pure form as the basis for a drug, whereas traditionally the whole plant was used which lessens the possibility of side effects.

In ancient times, the foxglove plant (*Digitalis purpurea*) was used for heart problems. In modern times, scientists have isolated the main active ingredient of the foxglove (digoxin) and put it into tablet form but in so doing have created a real risk of side effects. If the whole plant is used, the active ingredient interacts with all the other constituents of the plant which naturally includes 'buffer' ingredients that counteract any side effect. Herbalists believe this is the proper way to use the healing powers of herbs and plants.

What is the best way to take herbal medicine?

The easiest and most effective way to take herbs is in tincture form using approximately 5ml (1 teaspoon) three times daily in a little water. Try to get tinctures made from organically grown herbs. In liquid form the herbs are already dissolved and are absorbed faster so their action is quicker. In the dry form, the tablets or capsules have to be digested and the benefit of the herbs is only as good as your own digestive and absorption processes.

Herbs are not like drugs. If you stop taking drugs the symptoms can return and you are back where you started. The herbs stop the symptoms but also, at the same time, they address the cause of the problem so that the body becomes more balanced and the symptons will not return.

Aromatherapy

Aromatherapy has been popular for centuries. Egyptians used frankincense for embalming and Cleopatra was reputed to have seduced Mark Antony by wearing jasmine oil: perhaps one to try for an evening at home! Hippocrates, the father of medicine, stated that 'the way to good health is to take an aromatic bath and fragrant massage every day'. During both World Wars, clove, thyme and camomile oil were used as substitutes for scarce disinfectants.

Aromatherapy uses essential oils for many different things. It can help you with weight loss because there are oils which can alleviate mood and anxiety and help combat any feelings of self-deprivation.

The term 'aromatherapy' was used in the 1930s by the French chemist Rene Gattefosse. While working in a laboratory, he burned his hand and plunged it into a nearby bowl of lavender oil. The burn healed quickly with little scarring. This event prompted him to investigate the medicinal powers of pure essential oils which are found in the stem, flowers, leaves, bark, seeds or peel of aromatic plants. Once extracted, these become more concentrated and potent. Each essential oil has its own specific properties and works through our sense of smell and by being absorbed into the bloodstream via the skin and lungs (where it has a therapeutic effect on organs, glands and tissue). As an example, clary sage is wonderful for lifting moods and seems to be particularly effective blended with geranium.

Rules for using aromatherapy oils:

- The oils are volatile so must be kept in dark glass bottles out of the sun and at a cool temperature.
- If the essential oil is to come into contact with your skin it must be blended in a carrier oil, such as almond oil, or diluted in water (exceptions to this rule are lavender and tea tree oils).
- It's okay to use neat drops of oil in the bath.

There are a number of ways to use essential oils:

Massage is very popular as a way of targeting either problem areas or your whole body. If you bath or shower first it allows the oil to be better absorbed. Use 5 drops of essential oil to 10ml (2 teaspsoons) of carrier oil. If your skin is particularly sensitive use jojoba oil as your carrier. Do not use oil on broken or infected skin.

Baths or showers are ideal for enjoying aromatherapy oils. For a bath, add 5 drops of essential oil just before you step into the water so that the oil is strong. Don't have the water too hot or the oil will disperse too quickly. Make sure the room is warm and soak for 10-15 minutes, inhaling the steam as you soak. When showering use 5 drops of essential oil to 10ml (2 teasp-soons) of carrier oil and massage yourself using a mitt or sponge as you stand under the spray.

Footbaths are a gift to tired feet. Put 4 drops of essential oil directly into a bowl of warm water and soak your feet for 15-20 minutes.

Inhalation is a less common way of using oils but can be beneficial for headaches which you could experience as you begin to withdraw certain foods, like coffee, from your way of eating. Fill a basin with hot water, add 2-3 drops of essential oil directly into the water and make a tent over your head with a towel so that none of the aromatic steam escapes. Breathe deeply for five minutes, keeping your eyes closed.

Other ways to inhale essential oils:

- Place a few drops on a tissue or pillow.
- Add a few drops to a bowl of water and place near a radiator so that the oil vaporises.
- Add 8 drops to 300ml (½ pint)of water to use as a room spray.
- Use scented light bulb rings, essential oil burners and steam vaporisers.

HOMEOPATHY

The word homeopathy comes from the Greek words *omio* meaning 'same' and *pathos* meaning 'suffering'. It is a treatment of 'like with like' so that the person complaining of certain symptoms is given a homeopathic remedy which produces the same symptoms. Homeopathy was founded by Samuel Hahnemann, a German doctor, and is an extremely safe form of medicine. It helps the body to fight its own battles by prescribing remedies in minute amounts. It is in direct contrast to allopathic medicine (most Western medi-cine) which treats symptoms by trying to create the opposite effect from which the person is complaining. If a person is feeling very stressed, anxious and has palpitations, for example, a homeopathic remedy would actually create the same set of symptoms, thereby encouraging the body's own heal-ing mechanisms. Modern conventional medicine, on the other hand, would prescribe drugs such as tranquillizers and beta blockers to create calmness.

In homeopathy, different people may be prescribed different remedies for the same problem. Homeopaths take a very detailed history of the individual. They not only look at the symptoms the person is suffering from at that moment but also find out what they like and dislike, whether they are a hot or cold person, their personality characteristics, food cravings and also their physical type. Long standing problems such as an underactive thyroid are often treated constitutionally by homeopaths rather than just symptomatically. Homeopathy can also help with underlying emotional and psychological problems that may have led to over-eating in the first place.

Health food shops and some chemists sell homeopathic remedies and many of these will provide guidance; some even produce leaflets. Minor problems can be self-treated but more serious matters need the expert advice of a qualified homeopath (see the list of addresses on page 185)

ACUPUNCTURE

This ancient Chinese system of medicine which dates back some 2,000 years is based on the concept of Qi (pronounced 'chee') which roughly translated means a form of energy. The acupuncturist aims to influence this flow of Qi through channels in the body called meridians to balance the physical and mental aspects of a person. This is not a self-help system so you need to see a qualified acupuncturist (again see the list of addresses on page 185). Acupuncture can be very helpful as you begin to change your eating patterns. It can help to control appetite and reduce cravings.

If you have difficulty obtaining any of the supplements detailed in this chapter then please see 'Staying in touch' on page 192.

CHAPTER 8

Tests to help with weight loss

There is nothing more frustrating than sticking to a healthy eating plan only to find that the weight you hope to budge won't move. There are a number of tests available which can help determine what may be preventing a successful weight loss. These tests can give invaluable insight into understanding your body better and working through the problems that may be holding you back.

We will now look more closely at the test for food allergies which we touched on in Chapter 5. We will also look at tests which can reveal vitamin and mineral deficiencies and alert you to any excesses of toxic heavy metals along with a test to see just how well your digestive system is functioning. These tests can help assess which supplements you need to bring your body back into balance and optimum health and prevent problems in the future.

If you have difficulty finding a practitioner to carry out any of these tests please contact me either by telephone or letter (my contact details are given on page 192).

FOOD ALLERGIES

If you tried the hypo-allergenic diet outlined in Chapter 5 and successfully pinpointed the food you are allergic to, you are probably not only feeling better but are also losing weight more easily. If you found, however, that you got confused when you re-introduced foods, then a food allergy test would be useful for you.

If you prefer, you can save time and confusion by going straight to the tests without doing the hypo-allergenic diet. The choice is yours and relies to a large extent on how unwell you are feeling and how urgently you need help.

Food allergies can affect people in different ways but generally symptoms include bloating, water retention, aching joints, fatigue, stuffy nose, skin problems, migraine headaches, asthma, digestive problems and weight gain.

These are not life-threatening but can effect quality of life on a daily basis.

Fortunately, these kinds of allergies can now be identified by a simple blood test which you can take yourself at home called the ELISA IgG test.

ELISA IgG test

ELISA stands for Enzyme Linked Immuno-Sorbent Assay. This is a very sensitive way of testing for food allergies. When food is not being digested properly (see 'Leaky gut' on p.150) food particles can leak out into the bloodstream. Instead of the body seeing these particles as food, it views them as toxins and sends out IgG antibodies to cope with them. When there are too many, they clump together and get deposited in the body's soft tissues, for example in the joints, muscles, skin and brain. This can cause symptoms such as weight gain, fatigue, water retention, joint pain and inflammation, to name but a few.

The most common foods that are known to cause digestive problems include wheat, milk, eggs, nuts, beans, sugar, yeast, fruit, vegetables, meat, fish, rice, corn and other cereals.

By measuring the IgG antibody reaction to them it is possible to discover which should be avoided.

Blood test

The test comes as a special kit, is relatively pain-free and takes only a few moments to do. It contains a disposable lancet which automatically makes a tiny puncture in your finger tip and the blood is collected in the tube provided. If you prefer you can obtain a kit which enables your practice nurse or doctor to take a small quantity of blood. The blood sample is then sent to the laboratory and after it has been analysed you are sent an extensive personalised report outlining:

- Foods that are highly reactive for you, those that are borderline and those that don't cause a problem.
- Recommendations of how to implement food changes and how to reintroduce the reactive/borderline foods safely at a later date.

I have had excellent results with these tests and I am told one woman lost 6kg (13lb) in four weeks after following the test's recommendations. Others have reported significant reductions in their symptoms. This test is considered to be very reliable and has even been used to identify clinical problems. It has also had scientific research published on it which supports these findings.[1]

CANDIDA

If you read the candida symptoms in Chapter 5 and felt you may be suffering from some of them then you may benefit from a simple test. As with food allergies on p.148, this is also a finger-prick blood test and can be done in minutes at home. You could have both tests done on the one sample of blood or, if you feel both tests are unnecessary, you can be tested just for candida.

The laboratory will scrutinise your sample for IgG and IgM antibodies. IgM reveals whether the candida infection was active at the time the blood test was taken, while the presence of IgG antibodies shows that you have had the infection in the past. Even when candida has been brought under control, the IgG antibodies will stay raised for several months afterwards.

LEAKY GUT

Tracking down the foods to which you may be sensitive is only solving half the problem. Why has the problem developed in the first place? What happens when you re-introduce the offending foods? The answer lies in the state of your intestines, the gut, and its capacity to process food properly. Food allergies are often a symptom that all is not well with the gut.

This is very important because if your intestines are not functioning properly you may not be absorbing nutrients efficiently which means you can become deficient in vital vitamins and minerals. This test, conducted on urine, can check the state of your gut.

All food must be broken down by the digestive system, passed into the bloodstream or dealt with by the body's lymph system. If this doesn't happen properly the undigested food moves much more slowly through the digestive system and can ferment and putrefy.

Large spaces can develop between the cells in the gut wall and food molecules can then pass into the bloodstream. This is called leaky gut or intestinal permeability.

Initially it is important to stop eating the offending foods, which will help to alleviate the symptoms and make you feel better. Then, the whole environment of the gut needs to be healed, in order to get the intestinal bacteria back in balance again so that you can stay healthy and prevent the symptoms recurring.

Urine test

Only recently has this condition become widely recognised and this very effective non-invasive urine test is therefore relatively new. It can be done in your own home with a kit that is posted to you. Two urine samples are required: the first is a pre-test sample, then you drink a special liquid which contains two types of marker molecules, and six hours later the second urine sample is taken. When the samples are analysed, the number of each type of marker molecules detected by the laboratory will give a strong indication as to how permeable (i.e. how leaky) your gut is.

PERSONALISED SUPPLEMENT AND NUTRITIONAL QUESTIONNAIRE

Modern-day living can take its toll on all of us. Being stressed and constantly rushing around can often mean that, even when we wish to eat well, we often can't. We want to stick to the best wholefoods, prepared and cooked in the best ways, but demands made upon us by work and family often find us resorting to convenience, take-away, cafe and restaurant foods – all of which are likely to be deficient in vital vitamins and minerals.

Our health also depends on how well we absorb and digest the nutrients that we do get. Problems such as weight gain, lack of energy, insomnia, headaches, depression and mood swings can often be traced directly to nutritional deficiencies.

It is possible to have a personalised supplement and nutritional programme designed specifically for you by a registered nutritional therapist. The therapist asks you to complete a questionnaire which explores your lifestyle, symptoms and dietary profile. The vitamin and mineral levels present in your body are checked and assessed for deficiencies. The questionnaire takes no more than 20 minutes to fill in. Once the therapist has analysed your answers the results are sent to you in a detailed report which outlines which of the 12 vitamins (A, D, E, C, B1, B2, B3, B5, B6, B12, folic acid and biotin), the seven minerals (calcium, magnesium, zinc, manganese, chromium, selenium and iron) and the essential fatty acids you are deficient in.

You will be advised as to what quantities you need to take in supplement form to bring your body back into balance and optimum health. The report also includes dietary targets to help you function at your peak levels of energy and health.

Three months later you complete the questionnaire again. The second results are compared with the first, to see how your levels have changed, and your supplement programme is then adjusted accordingly.

Vitamins and minerals work in balance with one another. It is because of this that it is vital you take the right ones in the right amounts, in the right combination and at the right time.

Mineral analysis

If you have been yo-yo dieting or restricting your intake and variety of food it is likely that you are particularly deficient in valuable minerals. It is important that these deficiencies are corrected while you are getting your eating back to a healthy pattern. It usually takes only about three months to resume the balance.

Hair test

This is conducted on a piece of your hair which is sent to a laboratory for analysis. The test determines which minerals you are deficient in and whether excesses of any toxic heavy metals are present in your body.

It checks for calcium, magnesium, zinc, selenium, manganese, chromium and nickel. The toxic heavy metal checks include mercury, aluminium, lead, cadmium and arsenic. A personalised supplement programme is then specifically designed according to the needs of your own biochemical profile. The results are given to you in the form of a graph (see opposite) so you can see how far your levels differ from the norm.

This test can tell you a lot about what may be going on in your body. People with low levels of chromium could indicate problems in keeping the blood sugar balanced. Those with high calcium levels in their hair may indicate a high calcium turnover in the bone, suggesting they might have problems keeping their calcium levels stable.

In both these examples the mineral in question needed re-adjusting. After the results of the test, any deficiencies can be supplemented and action can be taken to reduce the levels of any heavy toxic metals. High levels of lead, for example, can be reduced by supplementing with antioxidants. Your hair can then be re-tested in three months' time to confirm that the levels are back to normal or to indicate whether the supplements need adjusting.

It is wise to have the hair test done in conjunction with the personal supplement and nutritional questionnaire. By comparing your biochemical and lifestyle results, a more comprehensive profile of your overall condition is achieved. Compare the charts opposite.

Results of hair mineral analysis test before treatment

(ALL RESULTS IN PARTS PER MILLION)

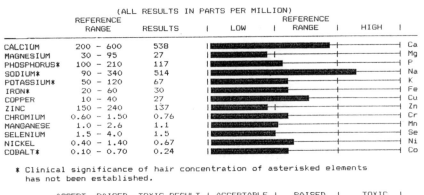

	REFERENCE RANGE	RESULTS		LOW		REFERENCE RANGE		HIGH		
CALCIUM	200 - 600	538								Ca
MAGNESIUM	30 - 95	27								Mg
PHOSPHORUS*	100 - 210	117								P
SODIUM*	90 - 340	514								Na
POTASSIUM*	50 - 120	67								K
IRON*	20 - 60	30								Fe
COPPER	10 - 40	27								Cu
ZINC	150 - 240	137								Zn
CHROMIUM	0.60 - 1.50	0.76								Cr
MANGANESE	1.0 - 2.6	1.1								Mn
SELENIUM	1.5 - 4.0	1.5								Se
NICKEL	0.40 - 1.40	0.67								Ni
COBALT*	0.10 - 0.70	0.24								Co

* Clinical significance of hair concentration of asterisked elements has not been established.

	ACCEPT	RAISED	TOXIC	RESULT		ACCEPTABLE		RAISED		TOXIC		
LEAD	<15.0	15.0 - 40.0	>40.0	4.1								Pb
MERCURY	<2.0	2.0 - 5.0	>5.0	0.37								Hg
CADMIUM	<0.5	0.5 - 2.0	>2.0	0.53								Cd
ARSENIC	<2.0	2.0 - 5.0	>5.0	0.24								As
ALUMINIUM	<10.0	10.0 - 25.0	>25.0	2.1								Al

Results of hair mineral analysis test after treatment

(ALL RESULTS IN PARTS PER MILLION)

	REFERENCE RANGE	RESULTS		LOW		REFERENCE RANGE		HIGH		
CALCIUM	200 - 600	516								Ca
MAGNESIUM	30 - 95	46								Mg
PHOSPHORUS*	100 - 210	170								P
SODIUM*	90 - 340	220								Na
POTASSIUM*	50 - 120	78								K
IRON*	20 - 60	21								Fe
COPPER	10 - 40	27								Cu
ZINC	150 - 240	193								Zn
CHROMIUM	0.60 - 1.50	0.71								Cr
MANGANESE	1.0 - 2.6	1.4								Mn
SELENIUM	1.5 - 4.0	2.2								Se
NICKEL	0.40 - 1.40	0.71								Ni
COBALT*	0.10 - 0.70	0.19								Co

* Clinical significance of hair concentration of asterisked elements has not been established.

	ACCEPT	RAISED	TOXIC	RESULT		ACCEPTABLE		RAISED		TOXIC		
LEAD	<15.0	15.0 - 40.0	>40.0	3.9								Pb
MERCURY	<2.0	2.0 - 5.0	>5.0	0.40								Hg
CADMIUM	<0.5	0.5 - 2.0	>2.0	0.17								Cd
ARSENIC	<2.0	2.0 - 5.0	>5.0	0.16								As
ALUMINIUM	<10.0	10.0 - 25.0	>25.0	1.6								Al

The two hair mineral analysis charts above show the difference before and after taking food supplements. In the first chart the patient has lower levels of magnesium, zinc and selenium, and her cadmium level is too high as a result of smoking. In the second chart, after following an appropriate supplement programme, her mineral levels are back to normal and the cadmium is reduced (she gave up smoking too).

CHAPTER 9

Meal plans for a week

Eat your way out of any diet

You will have learnt in Chapter 3 which foods to include in your new eating plan, but how do you put this into practice when you are feeding your family as well as yourself? The meal plans in this chapter assume that you will probably only be cooking for others once a day and able to choose your own food for breakfast and lunch. If you are at home during the week it makes the choice of food much easier, but many of us are at work during the day and our choice is restricted.

Most of us do not have much time for preparing meals, except when we have guests, so meals on a day-to-day basis need to be quick and easy to prepare and yet healthy and nutritious. The recipes I have given for the meal plans include quick and simple ones and those requiring more time. The recipes which have a variety of different ingredients can be adapted to suit how much time you have and what you have available in the cupboard.

Aim to keep the foundation of your food healthy so that when you are eating out it will not be a disaster if you include other less healthy foods.

I do not eat meat or chicken, so I have excluded these from the menus, but you are welcome to substitute these for fish in any of the appropriate recipes.

Give the old favourites a healthy boost

In your favourite dishes you can substitute wholemeal flour for white flour, free-range eggs for battery eggs, soya milk for animal milk and clear honey or maple syrup for sugar (weight for weight the same). Remember, if a food is described as 'sugar-free', this does not mean that it isn't sweet – look out for recipes made from naturally sweet ingredients instead of sugar.

If you suspect you may be allergic to wheat, you can substitute spelt for wheat in any recipes. Spelt is related to wheat but people who are normally allergic to gluten seem to tolerate it better.

I have included meals for a week with extra recipes for variations. If you are working and have limited choice of food for lunch, you could have sandwiches a couple of days a week and take something slightly more substantial on the others.

Sandwiches

Choose wholemeal bread. Wholemeal pitta can make a change from sliced bread.

Suggestions for fillings:
tahini and freshly sliced apple
hummous and salad
mashed avocado with a sprinkling of sunflower seeds
bean spouts and tahini
tofu mashed with a little miso and salad
tuna and salad
miso, tahini, lettuce and a squeeze of lemon
egg and cress
avocado and salads

Daily Menus

Monday
Breakfast – Choose a good sugar-free muesli and soak overnight in apple or orange juice
Lunch – Jacket potato with sweetcorn and salad
Dinner – Rainbow Trout (see p.162 for recipe)

Tuesday
Breakfast – Porridge oats: buy organic if possible and cook with water; top with linseeds or sunflower or sesame seeds, or mix in 5ml (1 teaspoon) of sugar-free jam or a dash of maple syrup. When using small seeds such as linseeds or sesame seeds, it is best to crack the seeds in a grinder or pestle and

mortar before you eat them, otherwise they can pass through you undigested. If you are constipated leave three quarters of the seeds whole
Lunch – Home made soup: try Spicy Carrot and Parsnip (see p.158 for recipe). Alternatively buy a tinned or fresh soup with good ingredients such as Baxters or Covent Garden
Dinner – Baked Cod (see p.166 for recipe)

Wednesday

Breakfast – Cornflakes: buy sugar-free cornflakes such as Lima or Doves' (usually sweetened with apple juice) and serve them with organic soya milk or organic cows' or goats' milk
Lunch – Smoked mackerel and salad
Dinner – Vegetable Lasagne (see p.165 for recipe) served with broccoli, sweetcorn (frozen is fine) and a salad

Thursday

Breakfast – Natural live yoghurt with your choice of fresh fruit: try bananas or strawberries
Lunch – Jacket potato with tuna and salad
Dinner – Fish cakes (see p.166 for recipe) served with Tasty Carrots and Parsnips (see p.158 for recipe) and salad

Friday

Breakfast – Dried fruit soaked overnight. When you buy dried fruit choose brands which do not have sulphur dioxide added. It is used to preserve the colour of apricots, for example, but they taste just as delicious without it.
Lunch – Sandwich
Dinner – Cheese and Onion Tart (see p.163 for recipe) served with salad and Sweet Potatoes (see p.163 for recipe)

Saturday

Breakfast – Wholemeal toast with sugar-free jam or marmalade. Avoid diabetic preserves which contain sorbitol; choose only those made with pure fruit such as Whole Earth, Meridian or St. Dalfour
Lunch – Tuna Fish Salad (see p.168 for recipe)
Dinner – Grilled Plaice with Tomato and Orange Sauce (see p.167 for recipe) served with salad

Sunday
Breakfast – Poached egg on wholemeal toast with grilled tomatoes and mushrooms. Use free range eggs
Lunch – Grilled Marinated Salmon Steaks (see p.171 for recipe) served with a
medley of mixed broccoli, carrots and sweetcorn and Curried Rice (see p.159
for recipe)
Dinner – Tofu Burgers (see p.173 for recipe) in wholewheat rolls with salad

Other Ideas

Breakfast
Grilled kipper with grilled tomatoes and mushrooms. Avoid artificially
coloured kippers.

Other suitable breakfast cereals: Shredded Wheat, Puffed Rice or Malted
Wheat Flakes with organic soya milk or organic cows' or goats' milk. Or
make your own breakfast cereal such as Crunchy Oat Cereal (see p.179 for
recipe)

Scrambled Tofu (see p.173 for recipe)

Rice

EASY WAYS TO COOK BROWN RICE

Brown rice provides more nutrients than white rice because it is a wholefood.
Use it in recipes where you would normally have used white rice.

BOILED BROWN RICE
Serves 2

250ml (8fl oz/1 cup) organic brown rice
475ml (16fl oz/2 cups) water
Pinch of sea salt

Wash the rice and place in a heavy saucepan. Add the water and salt, cover
with a lid and then bring to the boil. Once boiling, lower the heat and simmer for about 40 minutes or until the water has been absorbed.

BAKED BROWN RICE

The proportions are the same as for boiled rice (above) and I set it to cook for 1 hour in the oven 200°C (400°F/gas mark 6).

As variations on rice, try the recipes below:

BAKED RICE WITH HERBS
Serves 6

1 onion, finely chopped
1 garlic clove, crushed
15mls (1 tablespoon) extra virgin olive oil
175g (6oz) organic long grain brown rice
350ml (12fl oz/1½ cups) water or vegetable stock
2.5ml (½ teaspoon) basil
2.5ml (½ teaspoon) rosemary
Pinch of sea salt
1 bay leaf

Sauté the chopped onion and garlic in the oil until soft. Add the rice and stir until the rice is well coated with the oil. Stir in the remaining ingredients and bring to the boil.

Remove from the heat and place in an ovenproof dish with a tightly fitting lid and bake in a pre-heated oven at 190°C (375°F/gas mark 5) for approximately 20 minutes or until all the water is absorbed. Remove the bay leaf before serving.

SEAWEED RICE
Serves 4

225g (8oz) organic short grain brown rice
60ml (4 tablespoons) olive oil
2 medium onions, chopped
2 handfuls of arame seaweed soaked in water for 10 minutes and drained
30ml (2 tablespoons) tamari (wheat free soy sauce)
60ml (4 tablespoons) chopped parsley

Cook the rice in boiling water (twice as much water as rice) for 30-40 minutes until just tender. Heat the oil in a frying pan and sauté the onions until transparent without browning them. Crumble the arame, add to the onions and continue to cook for 10 minutes or until the seaweed is soft. Add the rice to the onions and mix in the tamari. When cool, add the parsley. Serve hot or cold.

(Recipe reproduced with the kind permission of Oliver's Wholefood Store in Kew Gardens.)

CURRIED RICE
Serves 4

225g (8oz) organic long grain brown rice
15ml (1 tablespoon) olive oil
1 onion, chopped
5ml (1 teaspoon) curry powder
50g (2oz) raisins
50g (2oz) blanched and chopped almonds (these can be bought ready for use in supermarkets)

Cook the rice as in the recipe for Boiled Brown Rice (p.157). While the rice is cooking, warm the oil in a frying pan and fry the onion for 4-5 minutes until soft. Add the curry powder and cook, stirring, for 1 minute. Add the raisins and almonds the stir well. When the rice is cooked, add to the onions and cook over a low heat for only 1-2 minutes to make sure everything is mixed well.

Soups

FRESH TOMATO SOUP
Serves 4–6

750g (1lb 10 oz) firm tomatoes
15ml (1 tablespoon) extra-virgin olive oil
1 large garlic clove, very finely chopped
A few sprigs of fresh basil, marjoram or parsley
750ml (1¼pints/3 cups) vegetable stock or water
Salt and freshly ground black pepper

Plunge the tomatoes into boiling water for about 15 seconds, then cool in running cold water. Peel and chop the tomatoes roughly, taking care not to lose any of the juice. Heat the oil gently in a saucepan and saute the tomatoes for a couple of minutes. Add the garlic and herbs and simmer with the lid off the pan for just 5 minutes. Put in the stock or water, salt and pepper, cover the pan and cook for a further 5 minutes only. To ensure a lovely fresh taste, do no overcook.

This soup can be served hot, but is even better chilled in summer.

SPICY CARROT AND PARSNIP SOUP
Serves 6

225g (8oz) carrots, chopped
450g (1lb) parsnips
1 onion, chopped
30ml (2 tablespoons) olive oil
15ml (1 tablespoon) curry powder
350ml (12fl oz/1½ cups) vegetable stock or water
300ml (½ pint) soya milk or organic milk
5ml (1teaspoon) sea salt
10ml (2 teaspoons) cumin seeds

If the carrots and parsnips are organic, then there is no need to peel them: just scrub them clean. Cut the parsnips in half and remove the woody centre. Cut both the parsnips and carrots into even-sized pieces.

Heat the oil in a heavy saucepan, add the vegetables and stir to coat in the oil. Add the curry powder and stir for 1 minute. Stir in the vegetable stock and milk and season to taste. Bring to the boil and then gently simmer for 20 minutes or until the vegetables are soft.

Blend the mixture in a food processor until smooth. Toast the cumin seeds by gently roasting in a frying pan without oil but stirring constantly. Use the seeds as a garnish.

This soup can also be made with pumpkin instead of carrots and also with any other mixture of root vegetables.

Main dishes and salads

GRILLED POLENTA WITH TOMATO AND CHILLI SAUCE AND BLACK BEAN CASSEROLE
Serves 4

For the Polenta
1 litre (1¾ pints/4 cups) water
225g (8oz) polenta
25g (1oz) butter
50g (2oz) strong vegetarian Cheddar, grated
30 ml (2 tablespoons) olive oil
For the Tomato and Chilli Sauce
1 small onion, finely chopped
2 cloves of garlic, crushed
1 tablespoon olive oil
1 dried ancho chilli, crushed, or 10ml (2 teaspoons) dried chilli flakes
225g (8oz) fresh plum tomatoes, peeled and chopped
10 ml (2 teaspoons) tomato purée
5ml (1 teaspoon) dried oregano
2.5ml (½ teaspoon) salt
Freshly ground black pepper
15g (½oz) butter
For the Black Bean Casserole
225g (8oz) black beans, soaked overnight
10 ml (2 teaspoons) cumin seeds
2 garlic cloves
5ml (1 teaspoon) salt
30 ml (2 tablespoons) olive oil

To make the polenta, bring the water to the boil in a medium saucepan, then pour the polenta into the water in a steady stream, stirring all the time with a wooden spoon. Continue cooking over a low heat, stirring more or less constantly, until the polenta comes away from the sides of the pan (20 minutes or so). Traditionally, the polenta is ready when a wooden spoon thrust into the centre stands up on its own without falling to one side. Add the butter and cheese towards the end of the cooking time. Grease a baking tray or dish with a little olive oil and pour the polenta in to a depth of 2cm (¾in). Smooth the top with a wet palette knife. Leave to cool.

To make the Tomato and Chilli Sauce, sauté the onion and garlic in the olive oil over medium heat until golden. Add the crushed chillies, tomatoes, tomato purée and dried oregano. Simmer for 30 minutes in a partially covered pan. Season to taste. Cool slightly, then blend in a liquidiser for a smooth consistency. Return to the pan and reheat gently. Beat in the butter in small pieces and simmer for another 5 minutes.

To make the Black Bean Casserole, cook the beans in fresh water and cover for about 1½ hours or until they are tender and most of the liquid has been absorbed. Meanwhile, toast the cumin seeds in a dry pan over medium heat until just golden. Grind the garlic, salt and toasted cumin seeds in a mortar until a smooth paste is formed. Stir the paste into the beans together with the olive oil.

When ready to cook, cut out shapes of polenta with a fluted biscuit cutter, brush with olive oil and grill on both sides under a hot grill until starting to brown. Alternatively, cook on the hob in a ridged pan. Serve on a pool of chilli sauce with the bean casserole on the side.

Note: you can use instant polenta, but to my mind it has a somewhat rubbery texture and is definitely inferior to the real thing. If you play some nice soothing music while you are stirring the polenta, the time passes quite quickly!

RAINBOW TROUT
Serves 4

4 × 175g (6oz) rainbow trout, cleaned
2 medium onions, chopped
5ml (1 teaspoon) sea salt
pinch of freshly ground pepper
250ml (8fl oz/1 cup) white wine
4 lemon wedges
sprigs of parsley

Preheat the oven to 180° (350°F/gas mark 4). After rinsing the trout under cold water, pat them dry and arrange them in a shallow baking dish. Sprinkle with the onions, salt and pepper. Pour the wine over the fish.

Bake for 20 minutes basting occasionally or until the fish flakes when tested with a fork.

Serve garnished with lemon wedges and parsley and accompanied with rice and vegetable and/or salad.

OVEN-ROASTED PUMPKIN
Serves 4

This can be enjoyed on its own or served with grilled fish, grains and salad. It goes particularly well with Watercress and Orange Salad (see page 169).

1kg (2¼lb) bright orange pumpkin
30 ml (2 tablespoons) extra-virgin olive oil
25ml (1 rounded tablespoon) rosemary leaves (fresh if possible)
Salt and freshly ground black pepper

Preheat the oven to 200°C (400°F/gas mark 6). Peel the pumpkin and cut into slices about 2cm (¾in) thick and roughly 8cm (3in) long. Put into a large bowl and drizzle with the olive oil. Toss to coat the pumpkin thoroughly, then sprinkle with rosemary, salt and pepper, mixing well.

Spread the pumpkin slices in a baking dish, making sure any rosemary leaves stuck in the bowl are transferred to the pumpkin. Bake for about 20 minutes, until the pumpkin is golden brown underneath, then turn and bake for a further 20 minutes or longer until the pumpkin is very tender and fragrant. Serve hot.

RED PEPPER AND TOMATO TERRINE
Serves 4

4 large red (or 2 red and 2 green) peppers
1 onion, finely chopped
2 garlic cloves, finely chopped
15ml (1 tablespoon) extra-virgin olive oil
750g (1lb 7oz) firm ripe tomatoes, peeled and chopped
Salt and freshly ground pepper
6 eggs, beaten
A few sprigs of fresh basil, chopped

Hold the preppers in metal tongs directly over a gas flame, or place them under a very hot grill or on a barbecue. Cook, turning frequently, until the skins turn black. This process should not take longer than 10 minutes, as you do not want the flesh to become too soft. Put the peppers in a plastic bag and refrigerate for 10 minutes. The skin will now peel off easily: this is best done under cold running water. Remove the stems, seeds and any membrane from the centre of the peppers and roughly chop.

Sauté the onion and garlic in the oil until soft. Add the chopped tomatoes and simmer for about 15 minutes with the pan uncovered, then add the peppers and cook for another 15 minutes. Season and cool slightly.

Add the eggs and basil, pour into a greased terrine or loaf tin and bake in a bain marie in a preheated oven at 180°C (350°F/gas mark 4) for about 45 minutes, until the mixture has set firmly. Unmould on to a plate and serve cool (but not too chilled).

ARMENIAN VEGETABLE CASSEROLE
Serves 4

This recipe can be made in large quantities and kept refrigerated. It's good hot, but equally delicious at room temperature as a salad. You can omit or replace some of the vegetables if like: pumpkin, giant white radish, parsnip, sweet potato or okra can all be used in this dish.

60ml (4 tablespoons) olive oil
1-2 leeks, sliced
2 potatoes, sliced
4 small carrots, cut into strips lengthways
4 medium onions, thickly sliced
2 courgettes, thickly sliced
2 red or green peppers, deseeded and cut into strips
1 small aubergine, peeled and sliced
4 large tomatoes, thickly sliced
Salt and freshly ground black pepper
For the Garlic-herb Mix
4 garlic cloves, finely chopped
100 ml (4 rounded tablespoons) chopped fresh herbs (including parsley, dill, fresh coriander, spring onions, celery tops)

Preheat the oven to 180°C (350°F/gas mark 4). Put a film of oil in a deep casserole dish. Combine the garlic and herbs in a small bowl. Layer the vegetables inside the dish and sprinkle each layer with seasoning, oil and Garlic-Herb Mix. Start with a layer of leeks, followed by potatoes, then the other vegetables, finishing with a layer of tomatoes so that their moisture will seep down through the rest of the vegetables during cooking. Drizzle over the rest of the oil, cover the dish securely and bake in the oven for 45–60 minutes, until the vegetables are tender but not mushy.

VEGETABLE LASAGNE
Serves 4

This is an excellent dish for serving up lentils to those who don't normally eat them. Seaweed is also used in this dish but in such a way that you can't taste it, yet you get all the valuable trace ingredients, so it is a very easy way of introducing it into the diet.

175g (6oz) brown lentils
5cm (2in) piece kombu seaweed
1 medium onion, sliced
1 garlic clove, crushed
15ml (1 tablespoon) olive oil
400g (14oz) can tomatoes
Pinch of mixed herbs
5ml (1 teaspoon) soy sauce
5ml (1 teaspoon) miso
15ml (1 tablespoon) Whole Earth tomato ketchup
1 packet wholemeal lasagne, cooked

In a pressure cooker or heavy saucepan with a lid, put the brown lentils together with the piece of kombu and enough water to cover. Cook until the lentils are soft, adding more water if necessary.

Lightly sauté the sliced onion with the garlic in the olive oil in a large frying pan or wok (you need a pan with slightly higher sides than a regular frying pan) until they are soft. Add the canned tomatoes and mixed herbs.

When the lentils are cooked, drain them, saving any excess cooking water, and add them to the tomato mixture. Keeping the heat low, stir well. Add the soy sauce, miso and ketchup. As you get used to cooking this dish, you can alter these last ingredients to suit your taste. Simmer for 5 minutes more.

Put the lentil mixture in a blender or liquidiser for just a short while with a little of the reserved lentil cooking water. This mixture forms the layers of the dish so it needs to be firm and not too runny.

In a rectangular baking dish, put one layer of pasta, then one layer of sauce and keep layering until the pasta is the top layer. You can add a sprinkling of grated cheese if desired.

Place in a preheated oven at 180°C (350°F/gas mark 4) until the pasta is slightly golden.

BAKED COD
Serves 4

1 medium onion, sliced
75ml (5 tablespoons) olive oil
550g (1lb 4oz) thick cod fillet, skinned and cut into pieces
3 large tomatoes, cut into wedges
30ml (2 tablespoons) capers
75g (3oz) black olives
30ml (2tablespoons) fresh chopped parsley

Preheat the oven to 200°C (400°F/gas mark 6).

Sauté the onion in just 15ml (1 tablespoon) of the olive oil until cooked and slightly brown.

Put the cod in a large baking tin with the tomatoes. Sprinkle over the onion, capers and olives and drizzle with the rest of the olive oil.

Bake for 20 minutes or until the fish is cooked (it should flake easily).

Sprinkle with the parsley and serve with brown rice (see page 157 for recipe)

FISH CAKES
Makes 12

550g (1lb 4oz) potatoes
225g (8oz) smoked haddock
60ml (4 tablespoons) soya milk
15ml (1tablespoon) lemon juice
30ml (2 tablespoons) fresh chopped parsley
sea salt and freshly ground pepper to taste
15ml (1 tablespoon) extra virgin olive oil

Boil the potatoes in lightly salted water for 20 minutes. While the potatoes are cooking, rest a plate over the boiling water and poach the fish in the soya milk. It is cooked when the flesh is firm. Mash the drained potatoes with the poaching soya milk. Add the flaked fish to the potatoes. Beat in the lemon juice and parsley and season to taste. Leave the mixture to cool.

Divide the mixture into 12 and shape into cakes about 1cm (½in) thick. Lightly oil a frying pan and fry the fish cakes for 5 minutes on each side.

TASTY CARROTS AND PARSNIPS

This recipe is so simple and yet so tasty! The quantities are quite vague so that you can design this dish to your taste, especially in terms of the garlic and ginger.

Carrots

Parsnips

5ml (1 teaspoon) extra virgin olive oil

Fresh root ginger, peeled and grated, to taste

Garlic, crushed, to taste

Tamari or soy sauce, to taste

5ml (1 teaspoon) maple syrup, or to taste

If the carrots and parsnips are organic, then leave the skins on; otherwise peel. Cut into wedges. Heat the oil in a wok and add in the ginger and garlic. Then add the vegetables and stir for a couple of minutes. Add 250ml (8fl oz/1 cup) of water, the soy sauce and maple syrup. Cover and cook for about 10 minutes until almost all the liquid has evaporated.

SWEET POTATOES

Serves 6

900g (2 lb) sweet potatoes

15ml (1 tablespoon) olive oil

150ml (¼ pint/⅔ cup) honey or maple syrup, or to taste

150ml (¼ pint/⅔ cup) orange juice

5ml (1 teaspoon) grated orange rind

Pinch of sea salt

Boil the potatoes in salted water for about 25 minutes until tender. Drain. Peel the potatoes when cool enough to touch and cut into quarters.

In a wok or large frying pan, warm the oil and then stir in the honey, orange juice and orange rind and bring to the boil. Add the potatoes and simmer, turning so that they are covered with the orange juice mixture.

CHEESE AND ONION TART
Serves 6

For a 23cm (9 in) pie crust:
175g (6oz) wholemeal pastry flour
Pinch of sea salt
75g (3oz) unhydrogenated margarine or 15-25ml (1-1½ tablespoons)
unrefined corn oil
about 45ml (3 tablespoons) cold water
For the filling:
2 onions, thinly sliced
15ml (1 tablespoon) olive oil
175g (6oz) organic cheddar cheese
3 free-range eggs
300ml (½ pint/1¼ cups) soya milk
5ml (1 teaspoon) sea salt
Pinch of ground nutmeg
Pinch of freshly ground pepper

Preheat the oven to 190°C (375°F/gas mark 5).

First make the pie crust. Mix the flour and salt in a large bowl. Add the margarine or oil and rub until like small breadcrumbs (or process in a food mixer). Add the water and mix with a fork until well blended. Roll out the dough on a lightly floured surface and use to line a 23cm (9in) pie dish. Trim away the excess dough and prick the pastry bottom with a fork.

To make the filling, sauté the onions in the olive until soft. Sprinkle the grated cheese in the uncooked pie crust and then place the onions on top. In a large bowl, beat the eggs and add the milk, salt, pepper and nutmeg. Beat the mixture together until well blended. Pour over the cheese and onions. Bake the tart for approximately 45 minutes until lightly browned.

TUNA FISH SALAD
Serves 4

15ml (1 tablespoon) cider vinegar
45ml (3 tablespoons) olive oil
5ml (1 teaspoon) mustard (optional)
Juice of ½ lemon
225g (8oz) cooked organic brown rice
200g (7oz) can tuna fish, drained

a few drops of soy sauce
5cm (2in) cucumber, finely chopped
15ml (1 tablespoon) chopped parsley

In a screw top jar, combine the vinegar, oil, mustard (if using) and lemon juice and then shake until mixed thoroughly.

Place the cooked rice in a large bowl and pour over the oil and vinegar mixture. Flake the tuna and add to the rice. Add the soy sauce, cucumber and parsley and mix thoroughly.

WATERCRESS AND ORANGE SALAD
Serves 2

1 large bunch of watercress
2 navel oranges
30ml (2 tablespoons) walnut halves, crushed
8-10 black olives (optional)
For the Dressing
Half a garlic clove, crushed
1.5ml (¼ teaspoon) salt
5ml (1 teaspoon) wholegrain mustard
Freshly ground black pepper
60ml (4 tablespoons) extra-virgin olive oil
15ml (1 tablespoon) balsamic or red wine vinegar

Wash the watercress in several changes of water, then pick over carefully, discarding any slightly yellowed leaves and the thick stems. Dry thoroughly. Slice the oranges, removing any pith and pips, then cut each slice into eight pieces.

To make the dressing, mash the garlic and salt with the back of a spoon to be sure the garlic is well crushed. Combine with the mustard, pepper, oil and vinegar. Just before serving, put the watercress, orange, walnuts and olives in a salad bowl, pour over the dressing and toss.

SQUID WITH ASIAN VINAIGRETTE
Serves 2

A refreshing meal of lightly cooked squid and crunchy vegetables with a tangy
Asian dressing.

500g (1¼lb) squid
100g (4oz) snow peas, blanched and halved
2 stalks celery, thinly sliced
2–3 shallots or half a mild onion, finely sliced
115g (4oz) sliced water chestnuts (fresh if possible)
For the Dressing
1 garlic clove, very finely minced
30 ml (2 tablespoons) rice vinegar
15ml (1 tablespoon) lemon juice
15ml (1 tablespoon) maple syrup or honey
5ml (1 teaspoon) soy sauce
2.5ml (½ teaspoon) Oriental sesame oil
2.5ml (½ teaspoon) salt
1.5ml (¼ teaspoon) white pepper
Chilli powder, to taste

Wash the squid thoroughly, peeling off and discarding the reddish-brown
skin. Pull the beaky part out of the centre of the tentacles and discard this, but
keep the tentacles. Cut the squid tube into pieces roughly 5x2cm (2x¾in).
Bring a pan of lightly salted water to the boil and put in the squid pieces and
tentacles. Simmer for about 2 minutes, just until the squid turns white and is
lightly cooked. Drain.

Combine all the dressing ingredients. Toss the squid with 30 ml (2 tablespoons) of dressing and refrigerate for 30 minutes.

Put the marinated squid and all the other ingredients into a serving bowl,
add the rest of the dressing and toss well. Serve lightly chilled.

GRILLED MARINATED SALMON STEAKS
Serves 4

4 salmon steaks, approximately 2.5cm (1in) thick
For the marinade:
15mls (1 tablespoon) per portion of fish, made up of equal parts soy sauce,
freshly grated ginger and freshly squeezed lemon juice

Pour the marinade over the salmon and let stand for 5 minutes. Turn the fish
over and leave for another 5 minutes. Remove from the marinade and grill
for about 3-5 minutes on one side. Turn the fish, brush with the marinade
and grill for another 3-5 minutes. Herbs such as sage or basil can also be sprin-
kled on top before grilling.

GRILLED PLAICE WITH TOMATO AND ORANGE SAUCE
Serves 4

4 plaice fillets
30ml (2 tablespoons) wholemeal flour
15-30ml (1-2 tablespoons) olive oil
For the sauce:
1 orange
350g (12oz) tomatoes, chopped
2 shallots, finely chopped
1 garlic clove, crushed
15ml (1 tablespoon) orange spread (sugar-free marmalade)

Coat each fillet with flour and drizzle about 1.5ml (¼ teaspoon) of oil on the
plaice. Grill for about 5 minutes until the fish is cooked.

To make the sauce, grate the orange rind and squeeze the juice. Put 30ml
(2 tablespoons) of the juice into a pan and stir in the tomatoes, shallots and
garlic. Cook over a medium heat for a few minutes. Stir in the orange spread
and, after bringing to the boil, simmer for about 20 minutes.

TOFU

Tofu is soya bean curd, made from yellow soya beans. On its own it has no
taste: its flavour is dependent on what you cook with it. It is very versatile
because of this ability to pick up the taste of whatever you combine it with
and because it can be prepared in a variety of ways. It can be sliced, cubed,

mashed, scrambled, puréed and used in both savoury and sweet dishes. So you can find tofu in soups, stir-fries, baked in casseroles, in dips, dressings, sauces and desserts.

Add tofu to an ordinary stir-fry simply by cutting it into cubes and cooking it with the other ingredients. Add strong flavours, such as garlic, ginger, tamari, etc., which the tofu will absorb.

My family prefer a very simple way of eating tofu. I cut it into thin slices rather than cubes and lightly fry it in olive oil. At the end of cooking when it is pale brown and the pan is still hot, I sprinkle the tofu with tamari and gently turn it over. It is eaten as it is, often simply with brown rice and vegetables, or used in sandwiches with mayonnaise, mustard and salad.

TOFU IN HOT PEPPER SAUCE WITH GREEN FETTUCINE AND SPINACH
Serves 4

500g (1¼lb) green fettucine
30ml (2 tablespoons) olive oil
500g (1¼lb) or 2 packets firm tofu, drained and pressed, each packet
cut in half
4 garlic cloves, crushed
2 medium onions, sliced
2.5ml (½ teaspoon) crushed dried chillies
600ml (1 pint/2½ cups) passata, smooth tomato sauce or tinned tomatoes,
whizzed in blender
Salt and freshly ground black pepper
1kg (2¼lb) fresh spinach
30ml (2 tablespoons) chopped flat-leaf parsley

Cook the fettucine according to the directions on the packet. Dried fettucine will take about 8 minutes, but fresh takes only 3 minutes or so.

Meanwhile, heat the olive oil in a large frying pan and cook the tofu on both sides until golden. I use a ridged pan and spray it with olive oil to cut down on fat. This way the tofu gets nice 'grilled' lines on it. Remove the tofu from the pan and keep warm. Add more oil to the pan if necessary and sauté the garlic, onions and chillies until the onions are tender.

Add the passata and seasoning, and simmer for about 8 minutes or until the sauce is hot and thickened.

Wash the spinach really well and cook in the water clinging to the leaves after washing. It will cook in approximately 3 minutes. Drain thoroughly, pressing down with the back of a spoon or a potato masher, and divide between four plates, making a neat mound in the centre of each. Surround with the fettucine, put the tofu on top of the spinach and spoon the sauce over the tofu. Garnish with the flat-leaf parsley.

SCRAMBLED TOFU WITH SWEETCORN
Serves 4

5ml (1 teaspoon) olive oil
225g (8oz) sweetcorn
225g (8oz) tofu, plain or smoked
10ml (2 teaspoons) soy sauce or tamari

Place the olive oil in a pan, then add the sweetcorn and the tofu crumbled into tiny pieces. Warm through by stir-frying and add the soy sauce to taste.

Arame seaweed can be added to this recipe: soak 60ml (4 tablespoons) in boiling water for 10 minutes or until soft, strain the water. The soaking water can be added to the mix when stir-frying.

(Recipe reproduced with the kind permission of Oliver's Wholefood Store in Kew Gardens.)

TOFU BURGERS
Serves 4

225g (8oz) tofu
1 celery stalk, very fined chopped
½ onion, very finely chopped
½ carrot, grated
Pinch of sea salt
50-75g (2-3oz) wholemeal flour
15ml (1 tablespoon) olive oil for each batch of frying

Drain the tofu and pat dry to remove excess moisture. Mash the tofu and mix with the other ingredients, except the oil. Use more or less flour to get the burgers to hold together easily. Heat the oil and fry two or three burgers at the same for approximately 5 minutes on each side.

SEAWEED

Seaweed is an excellent source of iodine which is vital in the healthy functioning of the thyroid gland which regulates metabolism. It makes up almost a quarter of the Japanese diet. There are a number of different varieties. Nori is the seaweed used by the Japanese to make a form of sushi (nori wrapped around rice with cucumber or fish in the middle). It is usually bought in sheets and toasted in the oven where it changes from brown to green. It can then be crumbled and used as a condiment to put on rice or pasta or added to soups. My family eat it cut up into squares: it is quite crisp once toasted.

Kombu, the Japanese equivalent of kelp, is very helpful in preventing the flatulence which can be caused by beans. Just cut off about 5cm (2in) – kombu comes in flat strips – and after discarding the soaking water from the beans, use the kombu in the cooking water. At the end of cooking, the kombu will be quite soft and you can break it up and eat it with the beans or remove it. Kombu helps to break down the starch molecules in beans which cause flatulence and you will also get the goodness from the kombu itself.

Agar is an easy introduction to seaweeds and I mainly use it to make desserts.

Desserts

Now you might be thinking that the savoury side of meal planning seems quite straightforward, but as sugar is not good for you, what are you going to do for desserts, cakes, etc.? You don't want to be deprived, but it means that you will rarely be able to buy cakes and desserts at the supermarket.

Healthy desserts can be very simple. Obviously fresh fruit salads, baked apples stuffed with nuts and raisins and live yoghurts are all easy options. You can also adapt recipes of ordinary desserts and cakes just by altering a few ingredients and this usually works out extremely well.

I make traditional desserts like apple pies and crumbles but just alter the ingredients slightly. Use eating apples instead of cooking apples, and then there is no need to add sugar (which is just empty calories). Raisins or sultanas can be also be added to give extra sweetness. For the pie crust and the crumble topping, I use wholemeal flour. I drizzle the crumble topping with maple syrup before it goes in the oven, which makes a lovely sweet crusty top.

MELON GRANITA
Serves 4

2kg (4½lb) ripe melons (such as rock melon, honeydew or cantaloupe, but
not watermelon)
10ml (2 teaspoons) orange-blossom water (optional)
Maple syrup if desired

Before you begin, turn the setting on your freezer to maximum. Peel the
melons and cut the flesh into chunks. Process a little at a time in a blender or
food processor to liquidise the flesh. Pour into a bowl, adding orange-
blossom water if using. Taste to check for sweetness; if your melon wasn't
fully ripe, you may want to add a touch of maple syrup (remembering that
chilling food diminishes the sweetness).

Carefully pour the mixture into icecube trays and freeze for around
5 hours until really firmly set. If you have several very small bowls, you may
like to put the additional melon pulp in these in the freezer rather than wait
until the first batch in the icecube trays is ready. If doing the freezing in stages,
store each frozen batch in a plastic bag or covered container in the freezer
while the next lot chills.

Process the deep-frozen melon, just a cupful of cubes at a time, in the
food processor until they turn into a sleety slush. Quickly put into a covered
container and store in the freezer while doing the next batch of frozen melon
cubes. When the whole lot has been processed, it can be stored for several
hours or even overnight in the freezer. Take the container out of the freezer
about 15 minutes before serving; if the weather is very hot, you may prefer
to leave it in the lower part of the refrigerator rather than on the kitchen work
surface before serving.

Spoon a little of the melon ice into glass bowls to serve.

ADUKI BEAN DESSERT
Serves 4

225g (8oz) aduki beans
600ml (1pint/2½ cups) unsweetened soya milk
Maple syrup or liquid honey
Sliced banana (optional)

Rinse the beans well and, if you've planned in advance, leave them to soak overnight. Otherwise, put them into a saucepan with 600ml (1 pint/2½ cups) of cold water, cover and bring to the boil. Simmer for 10 minutes, then let the beans stand with the pan still covered for up to 1 hour.

Drain the soaked beans well and put into a clean pan with the soya milk. Bring slowly to the boil, stirring, then lower the heat and simmer with the lid partially on the pan for 30 minutes. Taste the liquid (some brands of soya milk are already sweetened – these should be avoided) and add maple syrup to taste. Continue cooking until the beans are really soft and the liquid much reduced, adding a little water if necessary. The amount of time the beans will take to simmer depends on how long you have soaked them initially.

When the beans are soft, serve in small bowls, either hot or at room temperature. The beans can be refrigerated for 2-3 days, but be sure not to serve chilled or the flavour and texture will be spoiled. Top with sliced banana if you wish.

CRACKED WHEAT DESSERT
Serves 4

350ml (12 fl oz/1½ cups) burgul (bulgar) wheat
550ml (18fl oz/2¼ cups) hot water
6-8 dried apricots, chopped
30-45ml (2-3 tablespoons) raisins
120ml (4fl oz/½ cup) freshly squeezed orange juice
25g (1oz/¼ cup) walnut halves, roughly chopped
30-45ml (2-3 tablespoons) pine nuts, toasted in a dry pan until golden
Maple syrup or liquid honey, to taste

Put the burgul in a bowl and pour over the hot water, mixing thoroughly. Leave aside until all the liquid is absorbed and the grains have swollen. Fluff up the mixture with a fork.

While the burgul is soaking, combine the dried apricots and raisins with the orange juice and leave them until swollen.

Mix the burgul, dried fruit and nuts, then drizzle in maple syrup to taste. Serve at room temperature. You can serve this with some plain yoghurt if liked.

BAKED BANANAS

The essence of simplicity, this dessert of grilled bananas is full of flavour and natural sweetness. Of course, the bannanas taste even better done over a barbecue fire.

> 1-2 firm ripe bananas per person
> 5ml (1 teaspoon) sesame seeds per person
> A little ground cinnamon

Put the bananas, still in their skins, under a hot grill or over a barbecue fire and cook, turning frequently, until they are really soft when pierced with a skewer. This should take 10-15 minutes.

While the bananas are cooking, lightly toast the sesame seeds in a dry pan, shaking frequently, until they are golden brown. Turn into a small bowl, sprinkle with cinnamon and set aside.

Just before serving, peel the bananas and lay on a serving dish. Sprinkle over the sesame seeds and cinnamon mixture.

Lemon and Coconut Pancakes

> 115g (4oz) wholewheat, barley or rye flour
> 2 free-range eggs, beaten
> 200ml (7fl oz/¾ cup) Provamel organic soya milk
> 30ml (2 tablespoons) olive oil
> Juice of 2 lemons (buy unwaxed ones in the supermarket)
> Coconut milk
> 15ml (1 tablespoon) desiccated coconut

Sift the flour into a bowl, make a well in the middle and gradually beat in the eggs, soya milk and oil, either by hand or with a mixer. When smooth, leave to stand for 30 minutes. Heat a small frying pan and brush with oil. Drop in 30ml (2 tablespoons) of the batter, swill around and cook until bubbles rise and the underside is golden brown. Toss the pancake over and cook other side.

Put the lemon juice in a mixer with the coconut milk and desiccated coconut and blend. Roll up each pancake with a little sauce in the middle and pour some more sauce over the top of the pancake.

(Recipe reproduced with the kind permission of Olivers Wholefood Store in Kew Gardens.)

POACHED PEARS WITH CAROB CUSTARD
Serves 2

2 large pears
45ml (3 tablespoons) water
80ml (4 rounded tablespoons) rice flour
30ml (2 tablespoons) carob flour
750ml (1¼ pints/3 cups) soya or rice milk
Desiccated coconut, toasted to garnish

Peel, core and quarter the pears and simmer gently in the water until just cooked. Mix the rice flour and the carob flour with a little cold soya milk in a pan until smooth. Add the remaining milk and bring to the boil, stirring all the time. Simmer for 1 minute. Serve the pears with the carob custard and sprinkle with the coconut.

For a special treat, the custard can be made with cocoa powder and a little maple syrup.

(Recipe reproduced with the kind permission of Olivers Wholefood Store in Kew Gardens.)

APPLE CAKES
Makes 16 small cakes

450g (1lb) eating applies
225g (8oz) wholemeal flour
10ml (2 teaspoons) cream of tartar
15ml (1 teaspoon) baking soda
Pinch of sea salt
115g (4oz) unhydrogenated margarine
115g (4oz) honey or maple syrup
1 free-range egg

Preheat the oven to 200°C (400°F/gas mark 6) and grease a tray of patty tins. Cook the apples to a purée. Sift together the flour, cream of tartar, baking soda and salt. Cut the margarine into small pieces and rub this into the flour until the mixture resembles fine breadcrumbs. Stir in the honey and mix in the beaten egg to form a soft but manageable dough. Knead lightly on a floured surface and roll out 3mm (⅛in) thick. Cut out 16 bases and 16 lids.

Line each patty tin with a base, put in a spoons of the apple purée and put a lid on top. Bake for about 15 minutes.

BAKEWELL TARTS

These can be make as individual tarts or one big one.

Wholemeal pastry
For the filling
30ml (2 tablespoons) strawberry spread (sugar-free jam)
50g (2oz) unhydrogenated margarine
50g (2oz) honey
1 free-range egg, beaten
25g (1oz) ground almonds
1oz wholemeal self-raising flour
A few drops of almond essence
A few drops of vanilla essence

Preheat the oven to 180°C (350°F/gas mark 4). Line a baking dish or small individual tart tins with the pastry. Spread a layer of jam on top of the pastry filling. Blend all the other ingredients together and add on top of the jam. Bake until lightly brown and a knife when inserted comes out clean.

BREAKFAST

CRUNCHY OAT CEREAL
Serves 4

4 tablespoons clear honey or maple syrup
8 tablespoons corn oil
450g (1lb) porridge oats
100g (4oz) desiccated coconut
100g (4oz) raisins
100g (4oz) roasted nuts (almonds, cashews, peanuts, etc)

Combine the honey or maple syrup and oil and pour into a large bowl. Add the oats and coconut and combine well so that they are completely covered with the honey and oil mixture. Bake in a low oven for approximately an hour until hte oats are golden and cristp. Mix in the raisins and nuts and leave to cool, then store in an airtight jar.

Conclusion

This way of eating is not a 'quick fix' solution to your weight problem, but that is precisely why it works and why the weight stays off. Anything worthwhile is going to require some commitment and effort. When we learn any new skill it takes a few weeks before it becomes second nature and it is exactly the same with learning to eat differently. After a short while your new eating plan will be effortless and automatic.

When you lose weight too quickly it is just put back on again when you return to your old eating habits. As you change your eating patterns and lifestyle, watch the weight come off gradually and stay off..

You may have spent many years focusing on losing weight. If you make health your goal rather than weight loss, your whole perspective and relationship with food can change and so, automatically, will your weight. As Hippocrates said 'let food be thy medicine'.

Over a number of years, scientists have been looking at nutrition in a different light. They have realised that what we eat can have a role in the prevention of heart disease, cancer, osteoporosis, arthritus, diabetes, premature ageing and the treatment of many common conditions including acne, high blood pressure, infertility, irritable bowel syndrome and pre-menstrual syndrome.

Degenerative disease and illness is not inevitable. In other cultures, where people eat different foods, in different environments to us they are often free from our range of health problems. Yet if those people move to the West, or alternatively, if they adopt our lifestyle and diet into their culture then 'our' illnesses invariably start to appear.

As scientists learn more about the power of food, it is possible that Thomas Edison may be right when he said: 'The doctor of the future will give no medicine but will interest his patient in the case of the human frame, in diet and in the cause and prevention of disease'.

So persevere with making the lifestyle reccomendations in this book and see not only your weight change but also your health.

References

CHAPTER 1
Why diets don't work

1. Jeffrey RW et al., 'Does Weight Cycling Present a Health Risk?', *American Journal of Clinical Nutrition* (1996), 63 (Suppl), 452S-5S
2. Wynn A and Wynn M, *Journal of Nutritional and Environmental Medicine* (1995), 5, 41-3
3. Kreiger N et al., *American Journal of Epidemiology* (1982), 116, 141-8
4. Allaz AF et al., *International Journal of Eating Disorders* (1998), April, 23(3), 287-294)
5. Stenson, J, 'High-protein Diets may Defeat their Purpose', *Obesity* (1996), April 4, 8
6. Samaras K et al., 'Independent Genetic Factors Determine the Amount and Distribution of Fat in Women after the Menopause', *Journal of Clinical Endocrinology and Metabolism* (1997), 82-3, 781-85
7. Nelson M with Wernick S, *Strong Women Stay Slim* (Aurum Press, 1998)

CHAPTER 2
Mood, food and cravings

1. *Optimum Nutrition Journal* (1998), 11, 3, 16-21
2. Reproduced with the kind permission of Patrick Holford, author of *The 30 Day Fat Burner Diet*

CHAPTER 3
A way of life – not a diet

1. Feskanich D et al., *American Journal of Epidemiology* (1996), 143, 5, 472-479
2. *The Lancet* (1964), 2, 975-9
3. *Journal of the National Cancer Institute* (1985), 77, 5, 1053-61
4. Pearce ML and Dayton S, *The Lancet* (1971), I, 464
5. *The Lancet* (1994), 21 May
   The Times (1994), 24 May and 1 June
   International Herald Tribune (1994), 19 May
6. Reproduced with kind permission from *Now You Can Say Goodbye to Hydrogenated Fats* (1994), a leaflet supplied by Whole Earth Foods
7. The market leader for soya products in the UK is Provamel and as a company they

state that they are fully committed to producing foods that do not contain genetically modified soya beans

8. Coleman MP et al., *Trends in Cancer Incidence and Mortality* (Lyon, France, 1993, IARC Publication no. 121)

9. Ziegler J, 'Soybeans show promise in cancer prevention', *Journal of the National Cancer Institute* (1994), 86, 1666-7

10. Aldercreutz H et al., *The Lancet* (1992), 339,1233

11. Anderson J et al., 'Meta-analysis of the effects of soy protein intake on serum lipids', *New England Journal of Medicine* (1995) 333, 5, 276-282

12. Forsythe WA, 'Dietary protein, cholesterol and thyroxine: a proposed mechanism', *Journal of Nutritional Science and Vitaminology* (1990), 36 (suppl), S95-8

13. Albertazzi P et al., 'The Effect of Dietary Soy Supplementation on Hot Flushes', *Obstetrics and Gynaecology* (1998), 91, 1, 6-11

14. Gennari C, 'Introduction to the Symposium', *Bone Mineral* (1992), 19, S1-S2

15. Murkies A et al., 'Dietary Flour supplementation decreases post-menopausal hot flushes: effect of soy and wheat', *Maturitas* (1995), 21, 189-95

16. Cauley JA et al., 'Endogenous oestrogen levels and calcium intakes in postmenopausal women: relationships with cortical bone measures', *Journal of the American Medical Association*, 260, 3150-55

17. Severson RL et al., 'A prospective study of demographics, diet and prostate cancer among men of Janpanese ancestry in Hawaii', *Cancer Research* (1989), 49, 1857-60

18. Dr George Wald, Nobel Laureate in Medicine (1967), 'The Case Against Genetic Engineering' in *The Recombinant DNA Debate*, Jackson and Stich, eds. 127-9

19. Dr Mae-Wan Ho, *Genetic Engineering – Dream or Nightmare* (Gateway Books, 1998)

CHAPTER 6

Get moving – exercise matters

1. McArdle W, chapter in *Medical Applications of Clinical Nutrition* ed J Bland, (Keats, 1984)

2. *British Medical Journal* (1985), 291, 109

3. Bernstein L, *Journal of the National Cancer Institute* (1994), 86, 18

4. Kolner B et al., *Clinical Science* (1983), 64, 541-6
   Yester R and Martin R, *Postgraduate Medicine* (1984), 75, 147-9

5. Twomey T, *Patient Management* (1989), 29-34

CHAPTER 7

Still need more help with weight loss?

1. Leung L, 'Pantothenic acid as a weight-reduction agent, fasting without hunger, weakness and ketosis', *Medical Hypothesis* (1995), 44, 5, 403-5

2. Evans GW and Pouchnik DJ, 'Composition and Biological Activity of Chromium-Pyridine Carboxylate Complexes', *Journal of Inorganic Biochemistry* (1993), 49, 177-87

3. Langsjoen PH et al., *Drug Experimental and Clinical Research* (1985), XI, 8, 577
   Kamikawa T et al., *American Journal of Cardiology* (1985), 56, 247
   Yamagami Y et al., *Research Communication in Chemical Pathology and Pharmacology*

(1976), 14, 4, 721

Wilkinson EG et al., *Research Communication in Chemical and Clinical Pharmacology* (1975), 12, 1, 103

Kishimoto C et al., *Japanese Circulation Journal* (1984), 48, 12, 1358

4.   Van Gaal L et al., *Biomedical and Clinical Aspects of Coenzyme Q10* (1984), 4, 369

5.   Biochemical Journal (1990), 272, 1, 181-6

     Federation Proceedings (1985), 44, 1, 139-44

6.   Allegra C et al., *Clinical Therapy* (1981), 99, 507-13

7.   Racz-Kotilla E et al., *Planta Medica* (1974), 26, 212-17

8.   Nomura F et al., 'Liver function in moderate obesity – study in 534 moderately obese subjects among 4,613 male company employees', *International Journal of Obesity* (1986), 10, 349-54

9.   Hikon H et al., *Planta Medica* (1984), 50, 248-50

     Vogel G et al., (Arzneim-Forsch, 1975), 25, 179-85

     Wagner H in JL Bean and E Reinhard (eds) *Natural Products as Medicinal Agents* (1981)

10. Bendle A, 'The effect of konjac fibre on weight loss' (1991), paper held by Institute of Optimum Library and study mentioned in *The Optimum Nutrition Bible*, P Holford (Piatkus, 1997)

11. Stephens NG et al., *The Lancet* (1996), 347, 781-6

12. *Journal of the Institute for Optimum Nutrition* (summer 1996), vol. 9, no. 2

13. Knekt P, *International Journal of Epidemiology* (1988), 17, 281-6

14. Knekt P et al., *American Journal of Epidemiology* (1992), 127, 28-41

15. Comstock GW et al., *American Journal Clinical Nutrition* (1991), 53, 13-20

16. Palan PR et al., *Nutrition and Cancer* (1991), 15, 13-20

17. Gridley E et al, *American Journal of Epidemiology* (1992), 135, 1083-92

18   Christy CJ, *American Journal of Obstetrics* (1945), 50-84

     Rubenstein BB, *Federation Proceedings* (Federation of American Societies for Experimental Biology 1948), 7, 106

     Finkler RS, *Journal of Clinical Endocrinology and Metabolism* (1949), 9, 89-94

19   Hendler SS, *The Complete Guide to Anti-Ageing Nutrients* (Simon and Schuster 1985)

20   London RS et al., 'The effect of alpha-tocopherol on premenstrual symptomatology: a double blind study, II, Endocrine Correlates', *Journal of the American College of Nutrition* (1984), 3, 351-356

CHAPTER 8
Tests to help with weight loss

1.   Lene H, *European Journal of Allergy and Clinical Immunology* (1995), 26, 50

     Fell P et al., 'Annals of Allergy' (1988) presented at the 45th Annual Congress of the American College of Allergy and Immunology, California

     Hoj J, *Journal of Allergy and Clinical Immunology* (1996), 1, 3, 97

     Baker S, American College of Environmental Medicine, October 1994

Suggested further reading

General

Ho, Mae-Wan, *Genetic Engineering – Dream or Nightmare?* (Gateway Books, 1998)
Holford, Patrick, *The Optimum Nutrition Bible* (Piatkus, 1997)
Budd, Martin, *Low Blood Sugar* (Thorsons, 1994)
Sears, Barry, *Enter the Zone* (Regan Books 1995)
Nelson, Miriam with Wernick, S, *Strong Women Stay Slim* (Aurum Press, 1998)

Food and cooking

Cousins, Barbara, *Cooking Without* (Thorsons, 1997)
Lebrecht, Elbie, *Sugar Free Cooking* (Thorsons, 1994)

Any cookery books by Sara Brown and Delia Smith. Delia Smith uses good quantities of 'clean', fresh ingredients

Useful Contacts

Acupuncture
The British Acupuncture Council
Park House
206–208 Latimer Road
London W10 6RE
0181 964 0222

Homeopathy
Society of Homeopaths
2 Artizan Road
Northampton NN1 4HU
01602 21400
For a register of practioners send a large sae

Medical Herbalism
National Institute of Medical Herbalists
56 Longbrook Street
Exeter EX4 6AH
01392 426022
For a register of practioners send a large sae and a 29p stamp

National Osteoporosis Society
PO Box 10
Radstock
Bath BA3 3UB
01761 432472

The Nutri Centre
7 Park Crescent
London W1N 3HE
0171 436 5122

Nutritional Therapy
British Association of Nutritional Therapists
PO Box 17436
London SE13 7WT

Olivers Wholefood Store
5 Station Approach
Kew Gardens
Richmond
Surrey TW9 3QB
0181 948 3990

Staying in touch

TESTS, SUPPLEMENTS AND EXERCISE EQUIPMENT

If you are interested in obtaining any of the tests, supplements and exercise equipment mentioned in this book and find you cannot get them locally, then please send or call for a brochure which gives more details and explains how they can be obtained by post.

WORKSHOPS, CASSETTES AND VIDEOS

I occasionally give workshops or talks around the country and have produced cassettes and videos from some of these. Please call if you would like to find out more about future workshops and/or the recordings, and you will be sent an information pack.

CONSULTATIONS

If you feel you need to see and talk to someone personally, I am available for private consultations at the following clinics:

The Hale Clinic, Regents Park, London
Viveka, St Johns Wood, London
Liongate Clinic, Tunbridge Wells, Kent
Flint House, Lewes, East Sussex

For appointments and enquiries
Tel: 0990 329244 Fax: 0990 329255
Dr M Glenville
The Natural Practice, Danegate
Eridge Green, Tunbridge Wells, TN3 9JA

If you would like to hear more of my advice on any of the following subjects:

Natural Alternatives to Dieting
How to lose weight naturally
Natural Alternatives to HRT
How to stay healthy through the menopause and prevent osteoporosis
Natural Alternatives to Infertility
How to increase your chances of conceiving and preventing miscarriage
Then call: **0900 9800006**

Calls are charged at 50p per minute at all times. Helpline No. 0990 329244 (Standard national rate).

The Natural Practice Danegate Eridge Green Tunbridge Wells TN3 9JA